When asked for his opinion on the material in this book, Arthur L. Caplan, Director of the University of Pennsylvania Center for Bioethics, and sometimes called the "most quoted Bioethicist" in the country, told the author;

> *" you are most certainly correct that insurers set limits, ration, and absolutely decide coverage."*

> *And*

> *" You need to put it in the hands of patient advocate groups. JDF, Parkinson's, cancer, MDA etc. They can use these points to push health reform."*

Kimkris Publishing
P. O. Box 242
Nottingham, PA 19362

The Great Health Care Fraud
or
What Politicians Don't Want You to Know About Health Care

(How to Get Coverage Every Single Time)

Dedicated in memory of Sandra Lobb and in appreciation to Kim, Kris, Jeff and Angie, without whose help and understanding I would never have completed this book.

Author's Comment

While this book addresses a specific problem in the nation's health care system, it also provides an excellent example of what has gone so terribly wrong in America. Ever since the Reagan era, we have become a nation obsessed with making money the quick and easy way. And when I say money, I mean dollars, not progress and success as our parents and grandparents defined it. I mean liquid wealth that can be whisked off to a Swiss bank account, a foreign investment or some well hidden tax shelter. --- When I began work, ethics was what was fair and right. However, when I retired some 40 years later ethics had become what one can get away with, with the help of a very good attorney. Corporate managers are no longer driven by the need to serve and produce quality. They are driven by a need to extract ever larger bonuses off cleverly compiled short term statistics. Politicians are no longer driven by the needs of their constituents, but rather the demands of a privileged few. Investing in the stock market has become day-trading with super computers to the detriment of the American retiree. And, deliberate obfuscation and misrepresentation are now the ready tools of commerce. We have become a nation where the few are literally given license to mine the wealth of our forefathers outside the law, with complete disregard for ethics and with an insatiable appetite for more.

Viewed Within My Years

I've been so indestructible for all these many years,
and plowed a course right through so many others' fears.
I threw myself headlong at life so seldom looking back,
convinced desire could overcome whatever else I lacked.

This passion for the edge of life where strength could pull me through,
where try was simply all of me and all that I could do.
Hence I could change and mold this world to all I knew was right,
a sun that rose and never set horizons filled my sight.

Yet here I stand surprised and changed exchanging night for day,
so many miles still yet to go in what now seems my way.
The freedom from that rising sun now viewed in one more set,
horizons once ablaze with light now gray through all I've met.

Yet don't see this a lesser me the fire remains inside,
I still risk more than most deem safe to bail against the tide.
I've simply learned I can't do all and more what I should fear,
more centered in what can be done when viewed within my years.

Frank Lobb on turning 60

TABLE OF CONTENTS

I. Introduction

The legal definition for fraud is to knowingly deceive an individual for the purpose of intentionally damaging them. Unfortunately, that is exactly what the Conservative Wing of the Republicans Party is guilty of in their push to privatize Medicare (the Ryan Plan) and subject seniors to a health care rationing system that Conservatives have helped construct and hide from the American people. I can say this because I've personally contacted the likes of the Heritage Foundation, the AMA, U. S Senator John McCain, U. S. Representative Joe Pitts, Rush Limbaugh, Glenn Beck and so many others on this issue and been shocked by their acceptance of this affront to our sense of fairness and freedom. While decrying the evils of what they claim to be the seeds of future rationing in The Affordable Care Act (Obama-Care), these very same folks have shown themselves more than willing to defend the rationing that has been carefully hidden in state laws and given over to health care insurance companies. A system so carefully constructed and hidden that it took me ten years of hard work and multiple court actions to get to the truth. --- And there can be no greater proof of deliberate fraud than that each and every state has the exact same provision in their law. A provision drafted by the insurance industry. A provision that you have never heard of or would very likely never be allowed to see if not for this book. A book I guarantee the insurance industry and the Conservative Wing of the Republican Party don't want you to ever see. Language and provisions a Google search won't disclose and your doctor and hospital are barred from sharing with you. Language and provisions that sever the duty you would naturally believe your doctor and hospital owe you and your loved ones. ----

The purpose of this book, then, is to share what it took me ten years to uncover and, most important, to explain how to get the care you need from your private health care insurance policy every single time, ---- to insure you stay a step ahead of the provisions they have so carefully hidden from you, ---- to avoid the trap so carefully laid.

II. The Start of Our Education (The Death of Sandy)

We were a family like so many growing up in the 50's and 60's. Simply put, my wife Sandy and I were the product of small town America. In our case, that small town was Ridley Park, Pennsylvania. And like so many others in that period of history, we grew up sharing the same friends, schools, parties and events. Our parents were working middle class folks who belonged to the same church, regularly attended the meetings of the home and school association, never missed a football game and actively supported the town's many community activities. In short, we were an integral part of small-town America.

After graduating from high school, Sandy entered Drexel University where she majored in home economics. I chose engineering at Penn State. Following that, Sandy became a teacher at a local junior high school and I entered flight training for the US Navy. Five years later we were married in the Ridley Park Presbyterian Church with essentially the whole town in attendance. In short, life was good and our opportunities seemed endless.

What followed were three great kids (Kim, Kris and Jeff), my career as an engineer and then manager at DuPont, and our family life on a 200-acre farm located in Nottingham, Pennsylvania. Sandy was still teaching, although as a substitute teacher at the local Oxford Area High School. I was working for DuPont in Wilmington, Delaware, flying for the Naval Reserve out of NAS Willow Grove and operating our farm. And like so many couples of that time, we were far too

busy raising our kids and balancing the demands of an increasingly complex life to question the fairness of life or our country's institutions.

On the surface, we were a close and loving family enjoying a steadily growing slice of the American dream. However, as we all know too well, appearances can be deceiving and they certainly were in our case. Sandy became depressed over childhood issues I've never really understood. This depression led to excessive drinking and a dependence on alcohol that only grew with time. In short, we were transformed from a family who discussed everything to one that couldn't even acknowledge Sandy had a drinking problem. The kids and I slowly sank into a state of watching silently as their mother drank herself into a completely different person. We became increasingly dysfunctional and, to use a popular term in naval aviation, we were "spiraling in."

The problem only worsened with time and in 1990, Sandy and I divorced with the court giving me primary custodial custody of our three children. However, while the divorce was as bitter and painful as one can ever imagine, I managed to retain a reasonably close and cordial relationship with Sandy. She was a good person and it was important for the kids that we continued to have a close and supporting relationship. In fact, with the marriage out of the way, our relationship actually improved, even though I remarried. We met and spoke regularly and I continued to manage much of her affairs.

However, while some things improved with time, Sandy's health wasn't one of them. Her health remained a constant concern for the entire family. In fact, it became increasingly clear that her addiction to alcohol was likely to lead to the loss of her job and some form of physical and emotional collapse. And, since Sandy had never been willing to even acknowledge her alcoholism, it was generally agreed that this pending collapse would likely be our only chance to get Sandy the help she so desperately needed.

As fate would have it, Sandy's declining health and growing problems at work became so severe she was forced to ask for help. She literally phoned me out of the blue one night just to ask if I could help her find a doctor. She said she had known she had an alcohol problem for a long time, but had never been willing to deal with it. However, she was having so much trouble at school and her health was becoming such a problem that she really needed to find a doctor she could confide in. Someone who could provide the help she needed for her alcoholism.

Unfortunately, while I was able to put Sandy in touch with an excellent doctor, the help came too late. On July 26, 1997, Kris found her mother lying in bed in a state of complete collapse and near death. Kris immediately called the doctor who had Sandy rushed to the hospital.

The problem we faced was two-fold. First, Sandy's physical condition had deteriorated to the point where death was a real possibility. Second, if we were able to save her life, we still had to find a way to address the underlying alcoholism. Fortunately, Sandy's doctor and the hospital did a remarkable job in treating Sandy's many physical ailments. They literally pulled her back from death's doorstep. However, Sandy was still suffering from a significant degree of dementia, restricted mobility and of course her alcoholism.

To address these problems, the doctor prescribed a continuing program of physical therapy and in-patient alcohol rehabilitation. The hospital told us they were in full agreement. However, without any warning what so ever, I got a call from the hospital saying they were discharging Sandy and we were to make arrangements to pick her up that afternoon. When I asked "why",

they said Sandy's insurance company had determined she no longer needed hospitalization and the doctor was in full agreement. To say I was shocked is an extreme understatement. When I argued Sandy had never received the treatment for alcoholism her doctor was prescribing and she certainly was in no condition to be discharged, the hospital simply said their decision was final and we had no choice but to arrange to pick her up that afternoon.

I need to explain that while Sandy and I had divorced, I was still managing her affairs. Furthermore, I was still viewed as the head of the broader family unit that included Sandy. And while I lacked any legal standing to make decisions for Sandy, our oldest daughter, Kim, had a power of attorney and looked to me to make the right decisions.

While I am not an attorney, I'm also not ignorant on the law. My job at DuPont had given me years of experience in a number of areas of the law and I knew the hospital couldn't discharge Sandy without her doctor's concurrence. Furthermore, the doctor had reiterated strong support for continuing physical therapy and hospitalization for alcohol rehabilitation. In fact, I had just spoken with the doctor and she had again expressed that same opinion. Consequently, I demanded the hospital produce a recommendation for discharge signed by both Sandy's doctor and the hospital. This stopped things dead in their tracks and I honestly thought we had won. We seemed to have the law and Sandy's doctor on our side and, as best we could tell, all efforts to discharge Sandy had disappeared. Consequently, we naively assumed things were back on track and Sandy was getting the care she needed.

Unfortunately, three days later Kris noticed her mother wasn't being treated. She called me and after a few additional calls, I found Kris was absolutely right. The hospital had stopped all treatment and was ignoring the instructions of the doctor. In essence, Sandy was simply being housed and fed instead of treated for her numerous remaining problems.

I immediately called Sandy's doctor and got the following explanation. Sandy's insurer had stopped all coverage several days earlier and since then, the hospital had refused to provide any additional treatment or skilled care. Furthermore, the hospital was exerting increasing pressure to get the Doctor to approve discharging Sandy.

The doctor further explained that she had argued repeatedly with the hospital and Sandy's insurance company, but had hit an absolute brick wall. The insurance company was continuing to deny coverage and insisting the doctor agree to an immediate discharge. And without coverage, the hospital was refusing to provide any additional treatment. The doctor said she was at a complete loss on how to get Sandy the care she needed and both the insurance company and the hospital were exerting ever increasing pressure on her to discharge Sandy. Furthermore, since Sandy wasn't well enough to return home, the insurance company was insisting she be discharged to a nursing home where it would be impossible to get Sandy the care she needed. The doctor said she had even tried to get Sandy admitted to another hospital and been refused because the insurer was denying coverage.

Knowing the doctor was fully on our side, I demanded a meeting between our family, the doctor, the hospital and the insurance company. In a complete surprise to me at the time, the insurance company flatly refused to attend even though they had a representative resident in the hospital. However, knowing what I know now, their refusal should have come as no surprise. Had the insurance company attended the meeting, they would have had to witness the doctor prescribing "medically necessary" care for Sandy. By not attending, they remained free to characterize the Doctor's opinion as they saw fit. And in this case, they held, and have held to this day, that

Sandy's doctor fully agreed with their decision to terminate all treatment and discharge Sandy to a nursing home. In other words, by not attending the meeting, the insurance company remained free to misrepresent the entire situation.

The meeting at the hospital was one I shall never forget. Kim and I attended along with the doctor, and a representative from the hospital. The meeting began with the doctor and the representative for the hospital acknowledging Sandy needed additional treatment to "*achieve her full potential for recovery.*" The doctor's exact words. However, both the representative of the hospital and the doctor then said there was nothing they could do to get Sandy the care she needed because the insurance company was refusing to approve any form of additional care. In short, even though Sandy needed additional hospitalization, there was nothing they could do. The insurance company had denied every appeal the doctor and the hospital had made. Furthermore, the hospital was not being paid for Sandy's hospitalization and they were not in the business of providing free care.

Thus, we had come to where the rubber meets the road. As the old saying goes, "follow the money." There was full agreement that Sandy needed additional care, but the insurance company was refusing to pay for it. I responded as I would for any issue involving insurance. I attempted to separate the issue of what the insurer was willing to pay for from what needed to be done. I told the doctor and the hospital's representative that the insurance company's decision had nothing to do with caring for Sandy as I was willing to pay for whatever she needed. To which, now hold on to your seat, the hospital responded "they could not accept my money." I literally went through the roof. I demanded the right to pay. In fact I offered to write the check on the spot. I even went so far as to demand my right of contract under the US Constitution saying they had no ability to do anything but accept my money. As I said earlier, I'm not a lawyer, but I am not ignorant on the law either. Therefore, I didn't argue my right to pay, I demanded it! I argued that the hospital was a state-licensed facility and, as such, they had no right to refuse my money. As long as Sandy's doctor was prescribing the care Sandy needed, I had an absolute right to pay for and receive that care. The hospital's licensing requirements, as well as the State's health laws and their laws on consumer protection, guaranteed me that right.

Once again, for a brief moment, I thought we had won. Sandy would get the care she needed and I would fight with the insurance company at some later date. Unfortunately, this sense of winning was once again short lived. The representative of the hospital, in what I can only describe as a searching and uncomfortable voice, said the hospital's contract with the insurance company specifically barred them from allowing me to pay for Sandy's care. They were only allowed to accept payment from the insurance company. Consequently, I was asking the hospital to accept an open-ended cost to treat Sandy with no hope of ever getting paid. ---- Needless to say I was not convinced. So the hospital's representative offered to show me the hospital's billing records to prove they hadn't been paid a dime for Sandy's care since the day the insurance company first denied coverage and demanded her discharge. The representative said they couldn't even transfer Sandy to another hospital because the hospital would know in advance that there was no way to get paid. ---- I looked to the doctor for support and for the first time saw the doctor align with the hospital. The doctor said that, as unfortunate as it was, the contracts the doctor and the hospital had with Sandy's insurance company left no choice but to terminate care and discharge Sandy to a nursing home. Neither the doctor nor the hospital could allow me to pay for Sandy's care and neither could any other hospital. The doctor went on to say that this also meant she could no longer attend Sandy and would have to withdraw from the case.

The doctor said there was simply no way she could follow Sandy into a nursing home. And even if she could somehow arrange it, such a facility would have no ability to provide the care Sandy needed. --- In simple point of fact, we were not only being told that there was no way to get Sandy the care she needed, but that the doctor was "being forced" to withdraw from the case.

The hospital representative and the doctor literally pleaded with us to allow them to discharge Sandy. They said time and again that their contracts with the insurance company provided no other choice. And, they couldn't afford to treat Sandy for free.

Having hit the proverbial brick wall, Kim and I slowly and grudgingly accepted the discharge and agreed to look for another way to help Sandy. I honestly believed we could find some way to get her admitted to a different hospital that would allow us to pay for Sandy's care. Consequently, as the hospital was preparing Sandy for discharge, Kim, Kris and I jumped on the phone and conducted our own search for another hospital. We learned all too quickly that what we had heard in the meeting was spot on. Once the hospitals we contacted heard Sandy's insurer was denying coverage and we were offering to pay for her care, they literally couldn't terminate the call fast enough. There wasn't a single hospital willing to even discuss admitting Sandy. Unfortunately, by the time we reached this point, Sandy's discharge was so far along that there was no way to reverse the process.

An important thing to recognize about nursing homes is why Sandy's insurance company was so anxious to have her discharged to one. Nursing homes don't have the ability to provide skilled care and are little more than a boarding house for indigent residents. Consequently, there is no ability to charge any of the cost to the insurer under an HMO or managed care plan. Even better for the insurer, there is little or no ability to transfer a patient out of a nursing home to a skilled health care facility except for the most basic health care emergency. Sandy would be expected to live out her days in the home untreated and completely at our expense.

Well, if you haven't recognized it yet, we are not your normal family. From the moment Sandy entered the home, we began working to find a way to get her admitted to a facility that could provide the alcohol rehabilitation she needed. And while the home didn't have a resident doctor, they did have, as most do, a doctor that reviewed the condition of the residents on a regular basis. Working with him over the next several months, we were able to get him to formally prescribe admittance to an alcohol rehabilitation hospital. Of course, that made absolutely no difference to Sandy's insurance company. The doctor told us that the insurer was still refusing to cover any form of additional hospitalization or in-patient treatment for alcoholism even though Pennsylvania law specifically required them to cover 30 days of such care whenever it is prescribed by a properly licensed physician, as in our case.

However, by this point, the insurer's intransigence was no surprise. So we made a conscious decision to end-run the system by completely separating ourselves from Sandy's health insurance and pursuing the care she needed solely as private matter. We honestly believed that, so long as we never mentioned the name of Sandy's insurance company or raised the issue of coverage, we would have an absolute right to pay for whatever care Sandy needed. We just had to make it absolutely clear from our very first contact with the hospital that we would be paying for the cost of the care.

Using the prescription we had gotten from the nursing home's doctor, Kris phoned the admissions office of the facility he recommended and one we felt could provide the care Sandy needed. As I said, our plan was to completely separate ourselves from Sandy's insurance by

agreeing to pay for her care from the very first contact with the hospital. So, Kris never mentioned the name of Sandy's insurance company. She simply told them that Sandy's doctor had prescribed in-patient alcohol rehabilitation and the family would be paying for whatever care was needed. The hospital then explained that to qualify Sandy for admission, they would have to do an evaluation that would cost one hundred dollars. Kris agreed, and we sent the check confident we were making progress.

That confidence once again collapsed when Kris called to tell me the hospital was refusing to admit Sandy. Apparently they had determined she wasn't qualified for admission. Seeing red, I immediately called the admissions office of the hospital and heard exactly what Kris had heard. Their evaluation had determined Sandy wasn't qualified for admission. However, when I asked for a copy of the evaluation, the representative said "I am sorry, but we don't provide copies of our evaluations." My response was slow, deliberate and firm. I said that lady had a simple choice to make. She could agree to send me a copy of their evaluation or I would have it under a court order. I said I had paid her for the evaluation, I therefore owned it as a matter of law and the only choice she had was how I received my copy of it.

The woman's response was immediate and pleading. She said, *"Please, please don't do that. We don't really do an evaluation. We simply call your insurance company and if they refuse coverage, we refuse to admit the patient."* That is the only issue here.

I literally exploded into the phone stating that the insurance company had nothing to do with this admission. We had never even mentioned the name of the insurance company. The care Sandy needed had been properly prescribed and we were insisting on being allowed to pay for it ourselves.

In a clearly apologetic and pleading voice, the woman told me exactly what we had heard before. Their contract with Sandy's insurance company barred them from admitting any patient the insurer hadn't approved regardless of whether someone else was willing to pay for the care. Furthermore, they couldn't accept our money. ---- This was the policy of the hospital and there was nothing she could do to help us.

To simplify the rest of our story, Sandy eventually recovered to a point where she was able to return home and even go back to work. However, this was largely due to our strong family support and unwillingness to accept the outcome normally produced by a nursing home. Unfortunately, as good as it was to see the progress she made, Sandy never achieved her full potential for recovery. Her health had been so permanently damaged that any continued drinking could only lead to death. Worse yet, since she had never been treated for alcoholism, she was again denying she even had a problem. We were right back to where we were prior to her collapse. Not surprisingly, Sandy slid back into drinking and all we could do was watch. ---- A short time later, Sandy S. Lobb collapsed and died, never having received one day of the care her doctor and family sought to provide, even though we had repeatedly demanded the right to pay for every cent of that care.

What followed were five lawsuits and ten years of litigation aimed at uncovering the hidden maze of lies, state regulations and contractual provisions that allowed Sandy's health care insurance company to, not only refuse to provide the care Sandy's doctor demanded and Pennsylvania law mandates, but to also deny her family the right to pay for that care. Something I never would have believed possible if I hadn't experienced it first-hand.

III.   Our Naïve Pursuit of Justice

Sandy's death created an anger in me like nothing I can remember. The way she died and how the kids found her was clearly part of it, but there was much more. Her denial of necessary health care violated everything I had come to believe about this country. How could an insurance company have gained so much power? But also, how could so many people lie to us about what was happening? It contradicted everything I had ever learned about contract law, business ethics, common decency and our national sense of freedom. It simply wasn't part of our American way of life, --- certainly not as I had come to understand it!

In my mind, the only rational explanation for all this was that Sandy's insurance company had created practices that were well beyond anything the law allowed and were enforcing them through secrecy and pure economic power. Sandy's insurer was known to supply on the order of seventy percent of the revenue for the hospitals in the region. No hospital could stand against a customer with that kind of buying power. If such an insurer were to terminate its contract with a hospital, the hospital would be facing bankruptcy, for no business can survive the loss of seventy percent of its income.

In what would prove to be an all too naïve state of mind and an overly simplistic view of the problem, I really thought all we needed to do was to get the facts of Sandy's denial of care and her death into the open. And the best way to do that was to sue her insurance company. After all, the sheer weight of the evidence, along with the outrageous nature of the insurance company's actions, had to guarantee a win. More importantly, it would force state government to step in against the insurer and correct the problem for other subscribers.

Who could deny that we had been prevented from paying for Sandy's care and, given that, who could ever claim this was an acceptable practice for an insurance company? It appeared to be so simple. We just had to find an attorney and file the case. Unfortunately, I forgot two lessons an older gentleman had tried to teach me many years earlier. --- "Life is never simple" and "Life certainly isn't fair."

The first problem we faced came as a complete surprise. No one believed us. Attorneys literally laughed at our claim of being unable to pay for Sandy's care because there were secret contracts between Sandy's insurance company and the hospitals that forced them to refuse our money. Attorney after attorney turned us away without even looking at the case. And these weren't small firms or local attorneys. My years with DuPont and work with the U.S Environmental Protection Agency had given me a significant network of contacts in the legal profession. I also had two close attorney friends I could turn to for advice.

As with most things in life, persistence wins, and it eventually did for us. We found a large Philadelphia firm specializing in health care that gave every appearance of believing in our case and the issues it raised. That was the good news. The bad news was that they took our documentation and essentially disappeared for a year, all the while claiming to be researching our case in preparation for filing. However, just days before the statute of limitations would have expired; they dumped the case back in our laps with nothing more than *"we just don't think the case is large enough."* The attorney for the firm explained that their board had conducted a financial review of the firm's cases and decided to redirect their efforts to just a few large cases. He explained that our case just hadn't made the cut.

To say we were blindsided by the decision is an absolute understatement. Up until the moment of the call, there hadn't been the slightest hint of a problem. Furthermore, we had told the firm, right from the start, that our primary goal was to force the disclosure of what we saw as the outrageous practices of an out-of-control insurance company. And, while we had acknowledged the firm's need to profit from the case, we had clearly maintained that money wasn't what was driving us. Knowing this, they had taken an entire year to conclude there wasn't enough money in it for them. Furthermore, they coupled the rejection with a lecture on why our charges couldn't be true and, even if they were true, there was just "no" way we were ever going to get our hands on the contracts we would need to win the case. They argued the insurer's contracts were proprietary property that the insurer would never agree to surrender.

The meeting was so unreal that the attorney for the firm actually apologized for the message he was being forced to deliver. In fact, he claimed to be as surprised as we were by the decision and said he had argued the merits of our case with the head of the firm, to no avail. There was nothing he could do to help. --- Words we had heard all too often!

Aside from what I will always see as an outrageous breach of faith on the part of the law firm, their abrupt withdraw from the case left us without an attorney and with just days to go before the expiration of the statute of limitations for the case. They literally left us with less than a week to file a complaint or lose the right to ever file one. A task that, on its face, was impossible. How could we be expected to find new representation and have them file a major case in less than a week?

Knowing what I know now, I have to believe there was much more to this decision than the firm was willing to acknowledge. The scope of the issue we were raising and the reach of the insurance industry had to have played a role. Moreover, the timing of the firm's withdraw essentially guaranteed the case would be dropped. A clear win for the insurance industry and, as we would learn later, the industry's broad network of support.

For any normal family, this would have been the end of the story. It certainly should have been. But, not for the hardheaded Lobb family. Kim was the executer of Sandy's estate and, as such, could file *pro se'* for the estate. I, on the other hand, had enough experience with the law to draft a complaint. Consequently, I drafted a complaint and Kim filed it for the estate with a simple goal; we would preserve our right to pursue the case while continuing to search for new representation. Not for one moment did we ever consider pursuing the case essentially *pro se'* through five separate actions and years of lengthy filings and frustratingly complex responses.

Looking back, the effort was doomed from the start. First of all, we sued the wrong party. As I said, we were pursuing what we saw as the out of control practices of Sandy's insurance company, not a large financial award. In our mind, Sandy's doctor and the hospital were innocent parties that had done their best to get Sandy the care she needed. I also believed (again naïvely) that both were far more likely to testify to what happened if we left them out of the suit. After all, how could they testify to anything other than what actually happened if they weren't parties to the suit? I was so damned naïve! Even worse, I actually believed the court and state government would recoil on hearing what Sandy's insurance company had done. We even went so far as believing the court would provide a level playing field . --- So damn naïve!

So began what would eventually add up to almost ten years of painful and frustrating litigation (three actions in the state court system and two in federal court). All driven by the need to: 1.) Understand exactly how the insurer had denied us the right to pay for Sandy's care and 2.) Get

these practices disclosed to the public. Ten years of frustration and what the attorneys for Blue Cross, Aetna and the Commonwealth of Pennsylvania will readily describe as their success and our complete failure. However, success is always relative. It depends on the definition of what one is attempting to accomplish. In the case of Blue Cross, Aetna and the Commonwealth of Pennsylvania, their measure of success was having our cases dismissed by the court without ever having to address the underlying facts of their practices and contracts. On that score, they won every battle. However, our real goal was to learn how their system worked. On this score, our hardheaded persistence forced them to surrender, bit by bit, the full details of their system. Details we can now share with you and the public. ---- So, unless I am missing something, this is the win the Lobb family sought from the very beginning.

While the court records will never show us winning a single motion or hearing, this book provides all the proof the Lobb family will ever need for determining who actually won these cases. It discloses the details of a system that even the insurance industry cites as a violation of federal law, --- details that Blue Cross, Aetna and the Commonwealth of Pennsylvania demonstrated a willingness to do whatever was necessary to keep from us and you, the public, --- details that can insure you never face the denial of critical health care as we did with Sandy, --- details that can allow you to get the coverage you need <u>every single time</u>.

The records of all those court actions are available to anyone interested in following what I have already acknowledged were misdirected and frustratingly technical exchanges. Moreover, much of the language in that litigation is intentionally misleading because the defendants used multiple definitions for critical terms. In fact, it was a key element in their defense and success. Take for example, their use of the word "coverage". Because the care we had sought for Sandy was mandated by state law and clearly spelled out as an available benefit in Sandy's health care plan, her insurance company was forced to acknowledge that the care we had sought for Sandy was an "available benefit" under her health care plan, i.e., a *"Covered Service"*. However, in spite of this, the insurer used endless briefs, circuitous arguments, countless statements and completely misleading inferences to focus the litigation on whether we had been denied the right to pay for a *"Non-Covered Service"*. Try as we did, we were never able to get the litigation focused on whether we had been denied the right to pay for a *"Covered Service"*. The intuitive argument that the denial of a *"Covered Service"* automatically makes it a *"Non-Covered Service"* allowed the defendants to make sweeping statements about how counter intuitive, ridiculous and "frivolous" our suits were. After all, how could any responsible person argue that they had been denied the right to pay for their own health care?

In all those years of litigation, Sandy's insurer never departed from the subtle assertion that a *"Non-Covered Service"* includes any available benefit that they deny as not medically necessary or appropriate (see Exhibit #8). On the other hand, they also never stated it directly or in a way that they could be held accountable for what was and is completely untrue. They simply used these inferences to run us and the various courts in circles around issues that had nothing to do with the way Sandy had been denied care. And, for those who would question my earlier use of the word fraud, please note that the published definition for a *"Covered Service"* by Sandy's insurer is *"Covered Services"* are the *"services for which benefits are available"* --- the operative word being "available". Whether the insurer pays for a service in a particular case has nothing to do with whether it's a *"Covered Service"* (see Exhibits #6 & #7).

Simply put, for those who would choose to plow through the reams of paper that document ten years of misdirected and frustrating litigation, you need only access the readily available court

records of these cases. We will not provide that information here. From my perspective, all that litigation provides is striking proof of just how naïve we were in pursuing the various actions/suits.

All that being true, an even greater example of our naiveté was how surprised we were by the support and indifference we experienced for what we saw as the outrageous practices of Sandy's insurance company. We were literally Don Quixote with his lance and shield trotting out onto the field in defense of what everyone could only see as truth, justice and the American way! Unfortunately, the reality we faced was far different.

In my work at DuPont, I had led a number of efforts to interpret and revise federal and state regulations on environmental issues. That experience had taught me the importance of building a strong base of support for whatever you are pursuing. Consequently, while I labored with the mountains of paper thrown at us by the attorneys for insurers and the state, I was actively pleading our case to the likes of the Heritage Foundation, the American Medical Association, U.S. Senator John McCain, U.S Senator Arlen Spector, U.S Representative Joe Pitts, Pennsylvania State Senator Dominic Pileggi, Pennsylvania State Representative Art Hershey , radio and TV talk show host Michael Smerconish, Rush Limbaugh and a host of others. And while I certainly would never go so far as to say they were active supporters of the practices we were contesting, they certainly showed no particular interest in discussing them or disclosing them to the public.

Probably the most surprising one to me was the Heritage Foundation. This was an organization I thought would recoil at any interference with the right of an individual to contract in the private sector, let alone interference with an individual's right to pay for his or her own health care. Given the Foundation's mission and politics, I had expected them to jump to our defense. And they did at first. Their lead on health care, a Doctor Robert Moffit, spoke with me a number of times and gave every indication of full agreement on the right of an individual to pay for their own health care. He then asked me to document what we had learned so the Foundation could decide how it could help. That was the last time we talked or had any substantive contact. He simply acknowledged receipt of what I sent him and disappeared. Dr. Moffit and the Foundation literally dropped off the face of the earth as far as the Lobbs and this issue were concerned. There wasn't a single question or any form of follow-up on the information I sent them. Dr. Moffit and the Foundation simply vanished. In fact, I could only conclude they panicked when they saw the extent of the information I had collected. A conclusion that was reinforced by a warning I received from the Institute for Health Freedom. The president of that organization heard I had contacted Doctor Moffit and cautioned that the Heritage Foundation had a close relationship with Sandy's insurance company. While I can't speak to the accuracy of the warning, it certainly appeared to explain what I was seeing. In addition, a follow-up search on Google produced a number of articles by the Heritage Foundation defending the value of HMOs.

I had exactly the same experience with the American Medical Association (AMA). My first contact was with the Chester County Chapter of the AMA. In fact, I was asked to speak at one of their monthly meetings and received strong support for what they regularly saw as direct interference with their ability to treat patients. This support led to a letter of recommendation to the Pennsylvania Chapter of the AMA. However, just like in the case with the Heritage Foundation, all communication stopped. My attempts to follow up on the local chapter's letter of recommendation went unanswered. It was as if there was no one there.

Enter again the Institute for Health Freedom. I had been so disappointed by the unexpected turn of events that I mentioned it in a discussion with the Institute's president. She explained that I shouldn't be so surprised. The management of the AMA had a longstanding relationship with the insurance industry. While the local organization of the AMA was likely to show strong support for issues that directly affect the delivery of health care, the national organization is focused on its participation in managing the nation's health care system and the financial support it receives from the insurance industry. In fact, this financial support is to the tune of some millions of dollars. --- The message was clear. I was once again barking up the wrong tree. The national leadership of AMA wasn't interested in going to war with the insurance industry and the states. They were interested in maintaining their participation in the system.

Another surprise came directly from a U. S. Congressman. Our local businessmen's association had for some years invited state and federal politicians to speak at a yearly meeting to update local business leaders on the economy and government programs. One of those invited to speak was U.S Representative Joe Pitts. I had exchanged letters with Representative Pitts, but never succeeded in learning just where he stood on the hidden practices of the insurance companies. Consequently, I saw his attendance as an opportunity to question him directly. To say the experience was mind-numbing is an understatement. To his credit, Congressman Pitts responded directly to my question. And while he used a few more words than I will use here, he shrugged his shoulders and basically said that *"this is the system we have established and there is nothing to be done about it. Next question!"*

And lastly, there was one surprise I really need to describe to put into perspective the depth of support the insurance industry has for their ability to deny and ration care. In Pennsylvania, the law specifically states that insurance companies must provide up to 30 days of inpatient hospitalization for drug and alcohol rehabilitation whenever it's prescribed by a licensed physician. Exactly what we had sought for Sandy. Pennsylvania law also clearly states that insurance companies cannot override a doctor's decision in these matters.

However, because it had become so widely recognized that insurers were ignoring the law and denying coverage for the treatment of substance abuse, the Health and Human Services Committee for the Pennsylvania House of Representatives conducted a lengthy hearing on November 10, 2005, ostensibly to look into the matter. Appropriately, it was titled the "Hearing on the Impact of Denied Drug and Alcohol Treatment." I testified, along with a long list of others. Two of which testified to experiencing the very same problem we had experienced in trying to get help for Sandy. --- They had not only been denied the coverage due them under law, but, like us, they had been denied the right to pay for it outside the participation of their insurance company.

The first witness was a registered nurse who had sought inpatient drug rehabilitation for her 14-year-old daughter. She testified that after being repeatedly denied coverage for her daughter, she had pleaded with the hospital to allow her to pay for the care her daughter needed. Just like our experience with Sandy, the hospital refused to allow this mother to pay for the care. That night, after once again being denied care, the daughter kissed her mother good night, went upstairs and killed herself.

The second such witness was Jeffrey A. Thomas, a career professional in the field of substance abuse rehabilitation who had sought help for a member of his family. His resume´ read: *"Professional Credentials – Master's Degree in Human Services 1996, Licensed Professional*

Counselor since 2002, Certified Addictions Counselor since 1988 --- and Professional Experience – Worked in D/A inpatient since 1983 in positions such as Counselor/Therapist, Utilization Review/Admissions, Managed Care Contracting, Clinical Director and Administrator of a 180 bed facility."

Mr. Thomas testified that, after being repeatedly denied coverage by various agents for the insurance company, he discovered that the hospital was effectively barred from allowing him to pay for the care his family member needed. He testified that "*Had I not known the facility administrator personally and had she not agreed to help my family*" (by providing the care free of charge) we would have faced "*premature termination of care.*" He said there was just no way the hospital was going to allow the family to pay for the care needed and that the administrator had begged him not to file an official complaint because it would all too likely result in some form of serious reprisal against the hospital and him.

Mr. Thomas described in detail how the insurance company and its agents had run him in circles by deliberately manipulating the facts in the case. He testified "*I recognized this manipulation of facts as I had previously experienced it*" in my work with patients. This was essentially an exact repeat of testimony heard earlier from Linda Williams, a representative of the Pennsylvania Attorney General's Office. Ms. Williams had said "*Who among us has not experienced the exasperation of calling to verify coverage for a particular test or treatment, only to receive conflicting information from different customer service representatives on different occasions?*" --- "*The permutations are seemingly endless and inscrutable.*" --- It's as though they are speaking a "*different language*" or some "*code*" only known to them.

By this point, it should come as no surprise to learn that those holding the hearing exhibited absolutely no interest in following up with any of the witnesses or on anything they had heard. There wasn't a single question about how or why the witnesses had been refused the right to pay for their own health care, --- care that was mandated under law --- care that was properly prescribed by a state licensed physician. In fact, when I approached the chairman at the end of the Hearing, it seemed he couldn't separate himself from me fast enough. I got the old, "we'll be in touch." And of course, I never heard a thing. Just as my friend State Representative Art Hershey had attempted to warn me, the insurance companies in the state of Pennsylvania have the Legislature and its politicians locked up tight.

In summary, the Lobbs couldn't have been more naïve in their pursuit of justice. We filed against the wrong party, made the wrong charges, expected support where there was none and failed to recognize the importance of the issue to the insurance industry and government as a whole. We simply couldn't have been more wrong. We were the proverbial "babes in the woods" headed for slaughter!

IV. The Issue Unmasked (The Great Republican Fraud)

A. Getting A Copy of The Insurer's Secret Provider Contracts

From the moment we decided to sue, it was clear we were going to have to get a copy of what we had come to understand were the Provider Contracts that Sandy's insurance company had established with the hospitals that had refused to let us pay for Sandy's care. Most important, we would need a copy of the Provider Contract that Chester County Hospital had specifically told us prevented them from accepting our money.

Because Chester County Hospital had told us their Provider Contract was both required and approved by the State, we had to assume the contract was a public document and available to us as part of the general public. We further assumed that access had to be through the Department of Insurance for the Commonwealth of Pennsylvania. The only question was how and where.

Once again, my years of experience in state and federal regulatory affairs had me unusually well prepared to find the documents. And as is so often the case, the key to finding them and accessing them was to find someone in the system willing to help. However, unlike the documents I had accessed in my professional life, these Provider Contracts proved to be unusually difficult to find and access. In fact, I felt forced to conclude the State had deliberately created a "catch 22" to make accessing them all but impossible.

In order to see a copy of a Provider Contract, I had to know the document number under which the contract was filed. And, of course, it was state policy not to supply that information. I was just supposed to innately know the number. And, if by some quirk of fate I knew the number, I was assured I would be allowed to view the document.

One call led to another and then another and another until someone took pity on me and I had an invitation to visit the file room where the Department of Insurance kept its copy of the Provider Contracts issued in Pennsylvania. It was on an upper floor of the Department's facility at Strawberry Square in Harrisburg, Pennsylvania. I scheduled the visit, logged in and was escorted through a locked door to an assigned desk that I was told I could not leave without permission. It was like I was entering Fort Knox. I had to remain seated at the desk and could only review the material I was handed one document at a time. I could not photograph anything or make any copies. I even needed to get permission to leave the desk to go to the bathroom. However, the man overseeing me indicated I could make all the written notes I cared to write. And, most importantly, he handed me a copy of the master index listing all the names and document numbers they had on file.

This master index proved invaluable. It not only provided all the document numbers I needed to access the various contracts, it also listed the names of all hospitals under contract and the dates the contracts were executed. These dates were important because I saw immediately that the contract the Department had on file for Chester County Hospital was dated subsequent to the denial of care for Sandy. When I asked to see the earlier contract, I was told the Department only keeps a copy of the most recent contract. However, I was also told that I shouldn't be too concerned because the only real change in these contracts is billing rates. But probably the most surprising and significant thing I learned from the master index was that our doctor was also under contract to Sandy's insurer. In short, our doctor had essentially the very same Provider Contract with the insurance company as Chester County Hospital and the other hospitals that had refused our request to pay for Sandy's care.

Believing I wasn't allowed to make an actual copy of the contracts, I worked furiously to read them and take handwritten notes. A difficult task because these were long multipage documents and there seemed to be one for every doctor and hospital in the State. In fact,

there were multiple contracts for each doctor and hospital because each insurance company had its own Provider Contracts.

Obviously my reading and handwritten note-taking went on for hours. And then, out of the blue, my assigned monitor volunteered to mail me copies of what I needed. A bit too late as I had already completed my notes on all the pertinent Contracts. He said I just needed to pay a copying fee and fill out a request for each of the documents I wanted and he would see that I got a copy sent to me in the mail.

I will always believe that his offer to send me actual copies of the Provider Contracts I wanted to see was far more an effort to get rid of me than an offer to help. I was just taking too much of his time. And, after all, these were public documents and I had been approved to be there. Or at least he had every reason to believe that I had been approved to be there.

True to his word and not many days later, several large white envelopes arrived in the mail with letter perfect photocopies of the Provider Contracts I had requested. However, across the top of each cover-page in bold red lettering was the word "CONFIDENTIAL". In other words, these copies were not to be disclosed to the public or anyone other than me.

While these photocopies of actual Provider Contracts proved to be extremely helpful in pursuing our litigation; it has been the use of my handwritten notes from the Insurance Department's Library, open court records citing the actual language in these Contracts, state regulations, and a Provider Contract I was able to access on the internet that are solely responsible for the quoted material in this book and its Exhibits. I need to make this point absolutely clear, because I don't want to leave any room for a charge that the material in this book is protected under some state law or finding on proprietary information. If our 10 years of litigation taught me anything, it has been the willingness of the various insurance companies to do essentially everything and anything to keep these Provider Contracts hidden from subscribers and the public. That includes litigation and financial sanctions as a means of keeping the Contracts secret.

Yes, we eventually got copies of the pertinent Provider Contracts in Sandy's case through the discovery process. However, each was clearly labeled as proprietary information of the insurer. Furthermore, the insurer insisted that the court seal these copies so they could never be disclosed outside the case. Simply put, Sandy's insurer made sure the copies we received from the State and from the litigation process could never be shared with you or the general public. Unfortunately for them, the key provisions of these Provider Contracts are essentially universal and are available from sources outside their control if you know how and where to look and are as persistent as we have been. And, you don't have to know the exact language in these contracts to understand how they affect you. Not to mention that a strong argument can be made that federal law (ERISA) requires insurers to provide this information to their subscribers.

It's probably worth taking a moment to defend my characterization of the obstacles the insurance companies and the states have created to prevent subscribers from seeing the Provider Contracts that control a subscriber's access to necessary health care. I have met with far too many high-priced Philadelphia attorneys who told me very directly that I would never get my hands on a copy of these contracts. In fact, both the leading firm on

fraud, and the largest firm specializing in health care litigation in Pennsylvania, told us exactly that. --- To a man, these experienced attorneys claimed they had never seen an actual copy of a Provider Contract.

Looking back, it's clear, that if an attorney were to work long and hard enough, they could get a copy of a Provider Contract through the discovery process as we did. However, by that point in a case, an attorney will have spent a great deal of time and money and be effectively locked into a case. Given the fact that none of the attorneys we met believed we could have possibly been denied the ability to pay for Sandy's care, it's only reasonable that they would be reluctant to take a case like ours. Just like you, they would find what we were charging is far too counterintuitive to be credible. Remember, this type litigation is done on contingency. In other words, an attorney needs to have sufficient confidence in merits of a case before they can be expected to risk the time and money needed to assemble the facts in a case. And in our situation, they would have known that Sandy's insurance company would use every trick in the book to avoid releasing a copy of their Provider Contract.

The bottom line is that the state and the insurance industry have deliberately kept these Provider Contracts hidden from subscribers, the public and even the legal community. In fact, these Contracts contain strict confidentiality provisions that make it impossible for even your doctor and hospital to disclose the terms and conditions in the Contracts they have signed. And this has all been done in spite of the fact that these Provider Contracts are public documents that directly affect the care you and other subscribers will be allowed to receive. --- Out of sight, out of mind!

B. The Heart of The Fraud (The Enrollee Hold Harmless Clause)

While I could go on at great length about how one-sided we found these Provider Contracts to be, it would not serve the purpose of this book, as many of the provisions are aimed solely at the participating doctor or hospital. They don't directly effect a subscriber. However, for those who wish to delve into the detail of these agreements, they need only refer to Exhibit # 2 (a representative copy of the Provider Contracts retained by Insurance Department of the Commonwealth of Pennsylvania and other states, separate from any litigation and free and clear, with no strings attached). And while it is not, nor is it intended to be, an exact copy of any one insurer's Provider Contract, I can assure you it provides an accurate picture of the provisions that all insurance companies use to control a subscriber's access to health care. Fortunately, for those who would appreciate a simpler and more direct approach to these contracts, Provider Contracts can be summarized around seven universal provisions.

1. Every HMO insurance company licensed to do business in a state must establish a state approved Provider Contract with all the doctors and hospitals in their network of approved providers.

2. These Provider Contracts must include the "Enrollee Hold Harmless Clause" (Exhibit 1) as supplied by the state.

3. Insurers broaden the reach of their Provider Contracts by constructing them so that they cover all forms of insurance and apply to all of an insurer's subsidiaries and other affiliated entities.

4. <u>Most important!</u> --- The Contracts are structured so that they apply to all the products and services rendered to a subscriber, regardless of whether the insurer is willing to approve and pay for them in a particular instance.

5. <u>Furthermore,</u> --- Providers agree to: 1.) Accept and support the insurer's decision on Necessary and Appropriate care and 2.) Look only to the insurer for payment, including accepting non-payment as payment in full.

6. <u>However,</u> --- Providers must provide all *"Necessary and Appropriate"* care to subscribers, regardless of whether the insurer is willing to approve and pay for the care.

7. <u>AND,</u> --- Providers are barred from billing a subscriber or collecting from a subscriber except for charges associated with elective cosmetic procedures, experimental treatments, coinsurance and co-payments.

Points 5, 6 &7 form the very heart of the managed care business model. While a subscriber's coverage is defined as the benefits available under his or her plan, the insurer only has to pay for care that they alone decide is necessary and appropriate. In all other cases, providers agreed to render the care free of charge. Remember, to get coverage under an HMO/managed care plan, two things have to occur. First, the care must be an <u>available</u> benefit. And second, the insurer must <u>agree</u> the care is necessary and appropriate. However, neither of these two lessen a provider's obligation and duty to provide all necessary and appropriate care demanded by their license to practice and their professional responsibility. Simply put, in order to qualify for an insurer's business, providers must agree to provide all necessary and appropriate care, but to only get paid when the insurer agrees the care is needed and appropriate. It's the key to the insurance industry's power and their ability to ration and deny care. --- I trust there is no need to cite how reluctant doctors and hospitals are to working for free!

To understand these seven provisions is to breach a wall of secrecy that has been carefully set in place by the insurance industry and government. It also exposes exactly how the Republican proposals to privatize Medicare, the Ryan Plan and other such proposals, would subject all of us to a rationing system that already exists, is carefully constructed and ruthlessly enforced by the insurance industry. Rather than the rationing by government that Republicans claim will evolve from Obama-care, Republicans would subject everyone to an existing rationing system run by low-level insurance company bean counters that we will never see or even be allowed to speak to. --- Bean-counters that are paid to see that some percentage of us will never get the care we or our loved ones need, as in the case of Sandy.

For the Lobbs, gaining access to the State's library of Provider Contracts was the first time we were able to begin to understand exactly how we had been denied the ability to pay for Sandy's care. True, Chester County Hospital had told us their contract with Sandy's insurer had prevented them from accepting our money, but I honestly couldn't conceive how it could be done. After all, everything I knew about contracts and the law told me it wasn't possible. How could an insurance company deny us the right to pay for Sandy's care when we weren't parties to any such agreement? How could an insurance company establish contracts that were clearly in violation of so many laws, including the U. S. Constitution --- especially since we knew the contracts had to have been approved

by the State, i.e., the Insurance Department of the Commonwealth of Pennsylvania? And, how could one insurance company have gained so much power that they could deny us the right to pay for services that were available for sale in the open market?

While we began our pursuit of justice convinced that Sandy's insurance company could only be an out-of-control exception to the insurance industry, my visit to the State's library for Provider Contracts quickly put that misguided view to rest. There were Provider Contracts between every insurance company and with every hospital I had ever heard of. And while I couldn't be as certain about there being Contracts with all the doctors in Pennsylvania, the list of doctors under contract was so long that the same had to be essentially true for the doctors in the State.

One of the most interesting things was that all the Provider Contracts were pretty much the same. While there were the usual differences in language, terms, conditions and structure, the Contracts were remarkably similar. The only possible exception was the agreed-to-pricing that was not included in the copy retained by the State. Which raises an extremely interesting question: if these Provider Contracts are so similar and pricing is not included in the State's copy of the Contracts, why all the secrecy over a public document?

The one area in these Provider Contracts where there was absolutely no difference in language was a section typically titled "Enrollee Hold Harmless." Here, the Contracts were, word for word, the same. I can remember this being very striking to me at the time, because lawyers never use exactly the same language. I only learned later that the lawyers didn't have an option. The language was provided by the State and had to be included in every Provider Contract. It was and still is the law.

The following is the exact language of those Enrollee Hold Harmless provisions. It's also the language that complies with the requirements set-forth in the regulations of the Commonwealth of Pennsylvania and all the other states in the country (with the possible exception of Alaska) as well as the recommendations of the National Association of Insurance Commissioners. It's the language that must be included in the Provider Contracts that insurers are required to establish with every participating doctor and hospital in their network of approved providers.

Hospital/Doctor agrees that in no event, including but not limited to non-payment by Insure Company, Insurance Company's insolvency or breach of this agreement, shall Hospital, one of its subcontractors, or any of its employees or independent contractors bill, charge, collect a deposit from, seek compensation, remuneration or reimbursement from, or have any recourse against a Subscriber or persons other than the insurance company acting on behalf of Subscriber for Covered Services provided pursuant to this Agreement. This provision shall not prohibit the collection of coinsurance, co-payments or charges for Non-Covered Services. Hospital/Doctor further agrees that (1) this provision shall survive the termination of this Agreement regardless of the cause giving rise to termination and shall be construed to be for the benefit of the Subscribers, and that (2) this provision supersedes any oral or written contrary agreement now existing or hereafter entered into between Hospital/Doctor and Subscribers or persons acting on their behalf. Hospital/Doctor may not change, amend

or waive this provision without prior written consent of the Insurance Company. Any attempt to change, amend or waive this provision are void.

The really nice part about contract law is that the language in a private contract is held to mean exactly what it says. The only exception to this is where the language goes on to provide some narrowing of terms or requirements or there are exceptions specifically defined in the contract. Unfortunately for all of us, none of these exceptions apply here. Moreover, the language is mandated by law so exceptions or carve-outs aren't even possible. Simply stated, what you see is what it means!

Now, Pennsylvania, and almost certainly your state, will maintain that the intent of the language is not exactly what it appears to say. They will argue, as they have repeatedly done with me and throughout the litigation, that the wording is only intended to be a limited bar on balanced billing, i.e., a bar on providers billing an insurer and then billing the subscriber for the difference between the contracted price and the amount the provider actually wants for a service.

Unfortunately for Sandy and all subscribers of managed care insurance, what a state claims is the intended meaning of its language is of no importance when the language is included in a private contract. While the states are free to enforce the Clause essentially however they see fit, the courts have no such freedom when it comes to interpreting this same language in a private contract. The courts can only interpret a contract as it is written. After all, how can they view it any differently? Two independent private parties have agreed voluntarily to the language. Consequently, the courts have no choice but to accept it as written. So let's take a close look at the role the Enrollee Hold Harmless Clause plays in Provider Contracts and the denial of care for Sandy.

First and foremost, I need to say that without the presence of the Enrollee Hold Harmless Clause in the Provider Contract Sandy's insurance company had with Chester County Hospital, there would have been no need for all the litigation. We would have been able to pay for the care she needed and Sandy would almost certainly be alive today. Furthermore, if it wasn't for the fact that this very same Clause is in the Provider Contracts of all the other insurance companies across the country, there wouldn't be a need to write this book. In short, the Enrollee Hold Harmless Clause is at the very heart of what I am trying to expose through this book and what I believe is a deliberate fraud on subscribers and the American people. It's the engine that drives the insurance industries strangle hold on our politicians, our national health care system and our very lives. Again, it's the heart of a fraud that took me ten years to unravel.

To understand just how onerous the Enrollee Hold Harmless Clause is, one needs to have a clear understanding of the term *"Non-Covered Services"*. For if, as the insurance industry wants us all to believe, as well as every state regulator I have ever spoken with, the definition of a *"Non-Covered Services"* is any service that an insurer fails to approve and pay for, the Enrollee Hold Harmless Clause is essentially meaningless and we could have paid for Sandy's care. However, if a *"Covered Service"* is actually defined as: 1.) The *"health care service included in the benefit package"* (**Maryland Code Health-General Article 19-701**), --- 2.) The *"services and supplies for which benefits are available"* (**Glossary, Blue Cross Blue Shield**), --- 3.) *"the services/benefits specifically listed as included in a benefit package"* (**Affidavit of Howard W. McIntyre, Jr. in**

23

Exhibit #6), --- 4.) *"Defined by Aetna to be the services included in the policy benefit package"* (**Aetna written acknowledgement in Exhibit #7**), and --- 5.) *"Independent of whether Aetna pays for the care or denies coverage"* (**Aetna written acknowledgement in Exhibit #7**), then all these folks (the insurance industry and state government) can't be telling the truth.

Regardless of what you hear from your insurance company or your state insurance department, *"Covered Services"* are legally and contractually defined as the services contained in your benefit package regardless of whether your insurance company agrees to pay for them in a particular instance. Consequently, for all practical purposes, *"Non-Covered Services"* in HMO insurance plans and other managed health plans are limited to elective cosmetic procedures and experimental treatments, period! Remember, unlike indemnity insurance that spells out exactly what "is" covered under a particular policy, managed health plans (HMOs and other forms of managed care insurance) only spell out the care that is "not" covered by the plan. In essence, HMO insurance and other managed health plans essentially promise to provide all the care you will ever need except for elective cosmetic procedures and experimental treatments.

There is no better example of the insurance industry's willingness to deliberately mislead subscribers than their use of the term *"Covered Services."* For if *"Covered Services"* are the services available in a subscriber's benefit package, as they most certainly are, how can an insurance company claim to be *"denying coverage"* when they refuse to approve and pay for care that is clearly in a subscriber's benefit package, i.e., an available benefit? But that is exactly what insurers do when they refuse to pre-certify (approve) an available benefit. Consequently, they can only be deliberately trying to lead subscribers/you away from the fact that what they are actually doing is deciding you don't need the care your doctor is prescribing. They are directing the focus of the denial away from the fact that they are making a medical/treatment decision in direct violation of the law. Only a properly licensed physician or psychiatrist (your doctor) can prescribe care. Simply put, insurers are deliberately misleading the subscriber to keep their denial buried in the vagaries of insurance policies and procedures rather than a subscriber's rights under law. I will have more to say about these rights further along in the book, but for now, let's get back to analyzing the Enrollee Hold Harmless Clause.

Since we have established a clear definition for "Covered Services," we can say with certainty exactly what qualifies as a *"Non-Covered Service,"* as *"Non-Covered Services"* can only be those services that are NEVER available under a plan's defined benefit package. And unless your HMO plan or other managed health plan is uniquely different from the ones the rest of us have, those *"Non-Covered Services"* are limited to elective cosmetic procedures and experimental treatments. Consequently, the Enrollee Hold Harmless Clause's absolute bar on providers billing subscribers or collecting money from them for *"Covered Services"* has to apply to all forms of care except elective cosmetic procedures and experimental treatments. Once you know what a Non-Covered Service is, the Enrollee Hold Harmless Clause can't be read any other way!

But what if a subscriber simply agrees to pay a hospital separately as we tried to do for Sandy? In other words, the subscriber simply asks the hospital or doctor to make an exception and agree to accept a direct payment for the care required. Well, I need call your attention to the last two sentences in the Enrollee Hold Harmless Clause: "... ***this***

provision supersedes any oral or written contrary agreement now existing or hereafter entered into between Hospital/Doctor and Subscribers or persons acting on their behalf. Hospital/Doctor may not change, amend or waive this provision without prior written consent of the Insurance Company. Any attempt to change, amend or waive this provision are void." Here the hospital and doctor literally sign away their right to make any such agreement or any change to the Enrollee Hold Harmless Clause. And if you point to the wording that would appear to allow an insurer to "*waive this provision*" (the Enrollee Hold Harmless Clause) we are talking about waving language that is mandated in state law. In addition, the language specifically requires that any change be "*written*", completed "*prior*" to the rendering of care and formally approved by the state --- an impossible task. Consequently, there is just no way for a doctor or hospital working under the terms of the Enrollee Hold Harmless Clause to privately contract with a subscriber, agree to bill a subscriber or to collect from a subscriber for anything other than elective cosmetic procedures and experimental treatments. I've argued this point with countless attorneys and haven't lost yet. Please remember that the attorneys who wrote the NAIC's Enrollee Hold Harmless Clause were very smart people. Furthermore, they had to make the language airtight in order to avoid the possibility of subscribers being dragged into federal bankruptcy proceedings for insolvent HMSs. In short, there can be no holes in the language and there are none. The Enrollee Hold Harmless Clause is an absolute bar against subscribers self-paying for services contained in their benefit package or forming any type of direct contract with an approved provider that would in any way set aside the Enrollee Hold Harmless Clause's or its absolute bar against subscribers self-paying for services contained in their benefit package..

For those of you who may still question whether the ban on self-payment by subscribers is as absolute as I am describing it, we can look to how the courts are likely to interpret Provider Contracts along with their Enrollee Hold Harmless Clause. And while contract law in the United States is primarily determined by the various state legislatures, there are well settled elements that can provide the guidance we need.

First of all, there is general agreement that where contract language is clear and explicit, a court will ascertain contractual intent from the written provisions of the contract and go no further. Clearly, the language contained in the Enrollee Hold Harmless Clause is extremely clear and explicit. It states unequivocally that a provider can't bill a subscriber or collect money from a subscriber for services provided under the agreement (the Provider Contract). The only relief allowed is for the collection of coinsurance, copayments or charges for Non-Covered Services. Consequently, the only question left somewhat open for debate is the nature of a Non-Covered Service. However, we have already covered this point extensively. Moreover, a reading of Exhibit #7 will readily show Aetna agreeing with our analysis. Non-Covered Services can be no more than elective cosmetic procedures and experimental treatments.

Another point of general agreement on interpreting contracts is that technical words like "Covered Services" and "Non-Covered Services" must be interpreted as usually understood by persons in the profession. Again, a reading of Exhibit #6 fully resolves this issue. "Covered Services" as used by the insurance industry, regardless of what they might imply to a subscriber, are the services defined as available in a subscriber's benefit package. We can look to the following for additional corroboration, --- a Covered Service

is: 1.) The *"health care service included in the benefit package"* (**Maryland Code Health-General Article 19-701**), --- 2.) The *"services and supplies for which benefits are available"* (**Glossary, Blue Cross Blue Shield**), --- 3.) *"Defined by Aetna to be the services included in the policy benefit package"* (**Aetna written acknowledgement in Exhibit #7**), and --- 4.) *"Independent of whether Aetna pays for the care or denies coverage"* (**Aetna written acknowledgement in Exhibit #7**). And of course, our experience with Sandy provides the icing on the cake! Alcohol Rehabilitation was a mandated "Covered Service" under Pennsylvania law. Consequently, the fact that Sandy's insurer refused to cover the care did not and could not under law make that care a Non-Covered Service.

An additional point of general agreement is that contracts must be interpreted as a whole. Here again, there can be no support for an argument that the Enrollee Hold Harmless Clause is a limited ban on subscribers paying for Covered Services. All the Provider Contracts I have read state numerous conditions under which a provider *"shall not charge either the insurer or the subscriber."* These conditions typically include a failure to pre-certify the care provided to a subscriber, providing care not prescribed by a properly licensed physician, providing care that the insurer determined is not medically necessary or appropriate, rendering care that the insurer later determines is not medically necessary or appropriate, and failing to properly bill the insurer within 90 days of rendering care. All of these conditions providing for an absolute bar to billing the subscriber (see Exhibit #2). Consequently, even when taken as a whole, there can be no question that the intent of the Enrollee Hold Harmless Clause and the Provider Contract is to establish specific conditions under which a provider can NOT, under any circumstances, bill a subscriber.

And lastly, we will put to rest any claim that an insurer has the right to waive or relax this absolute bar on a subscriber self-paying for his or her own necessary health care. While the last sentence in the Enrollee Hold Harmless Clause clearly states that a provider *"may not change, amend or waive this provision without prior written consent of the Insurer"*, the statement does not provide the insurer with the authority to change, amend or waive anything. Consider the following: 1.) The *"provision"* referenced to can only be the Enrollee Hold Harmless Clause; 2.) The language of the Enrollee Hold Harmless Clause is mandated in state law; 3.) A change in the "provision" can only constitute a change in both the Enrollee Hold Harmless Clause and the insurer's Provider Contract; 4.) Any change to both a Provider Contract and the Enrollee Hold Harmless Clause will require some form of formal state approval, and; 5.) Any state approval to waive the language in an individual case would establish a precedent that would effectively invalidate the entire purpose of the Enrollee Hold Harmless Clause.

So, now that we have a clear understanding of Non-Covered Services and the Enrollee Hold Harmless Clause, is there anyone among us that isn't shocked by this secret ban on an individual's right to pay for their own, or their loved-one's, necessary health care? A secret that literally allows an insurance company to bar you from paying for care you might need to save your life or the life of a loved one, even if you can afford to pay for it. Remember, the issue isn't actually paying for care. In most cases we can't afford to pay for it. That's why we carry insurance. However, without the right to pay, we give our health care insurer the power to determine the care we will be <u>allowed to receive</u>, as in Sandy's case. We strip ourselves of the right to save our very life and the lives of our

loved ones whenever our insurer decides to deny coverage in pursuit of a stronger bottom line. Ask yourself, how can a hospital publish your patient's rights without disclosing that the Enrollee Hold Harmless Clause *"supersedes any oral or written"* agreement a patient thinks he or she has with their choice of a hospital? And, how can that professionally published pamphlet on patients' rights so prominently displayed in your doctor's waiting room not tell you that your doctor is under contract to your insurance company and has agreed to accept and support the insurer's decisions on necessary and appropriate care? Moreover, how can your employer subject you to a health care plan that has you surrendering your "right" to access necessary care without ever informing you? --- That is, unless they all have something to hide. What do you think?

In summary, under the Enrollee Hold Harmless Clause, doctors and hospitals can only bill you and collect your money for *"coinsurance, co-payments and charges for "Non-Covered Services."*--- *"Non-Covered Services"* being defined as any care for which benefits (payment) is <u>not</u> available under any circumstances. Consequently, these doctors and hospitals are completely barred from ever billing you or collecting your money for any product or service that is defined as an "available" benefit in your plan, PERIOD!

While I will say time and again that I am not an attorney, I can assure you that I have had many in-depth discussions with countless attorneys on the meaning of Enrollee Hold Harmless Clause and not lost a single one of these since I got to the bottom of what I will readily agree is a masterfully constructed fraud on subscribers and the American people. In fact, I just recently had one such discussion with an attorney whose entire practice is centered on health insurance in Philadelphia. He came at me time and again disputing my analysis of the Enrollee Hold Harmless Clause and applicable law only to end the discussion with *"I can't say I disagree with you."*

C. The Proof of Fraud

Throughout our five suits and ten years of litigation, we repeatedly asked Sandy's insurance company and the Pennsylvania Department of Insurance to explain how a subscriber can pay for health care given the language of the Enrollee Hold Harmless Clause. In other words, if the hospital or our doctor isn't free to bill us or take our money, how can we pay them when our insurer refuses to pay? In my mind, it's a very simple question. However, we never even came close to getting an answer. What we got was: 1.) Ridicule for asking the question when the answer is so obvious; 2.) There is nothing in the insurer's policy that would in any way interfere with a subscriber's right to pay for their own health care, and; 3.) The intent of the Enrollee Hold Harmless Clause is to prevent providers from balance billing subscribers. In fact, the replies were so well married I had to conclude they were using the same hymn book and had had a great deal of practice.

The first response was clearly an attempt to deflect our question. Never mind that as a subscriber we had both a customer's right and a legal right to an answer. The Federal ERISA law requires insurers to fully explain their plans. Even more to the point, all either of the two insurance companies we sued or the Commonwealth of Pennsylvania had to do to get the court to dismiss any of our cases was to explain how we could have paid the hospitals where we attempted to get help for Sandy. In fact, they could have simply blamed the hospitals for not taking our money and the cases would have been

dismissed. There would have been one short suit, not five lengthy actions. But, oh no, Sandy's insurer and the State thought it far better to drag us through ten years of litigation rather than to ever directly address our question of "how we could we have paid the hospital for Sandy's care."

Their second response was simply another attempt to deflect our question because the Enrollee Hold Harmless Clause isn't in a subscriber's policy. It's in the insurer's "Provider Contract" (a document the insurance companies and the State did everything possible to keep us from seeing and questioning). I can't begin to count the number of times Sandy's insurer and the State assured the court that there was nothing in Sandy's policy that could have possibly prevented us from paying for Sandy's care. Never mind that we never asked about Sandy's policy or our freedom to pay. We were asking about the insurance company's Provider Contracts and the hospitals' ability to bill us and accept our payment.

It's worth noting that the ERISA Preemption Manual for State Health Policy Matters published by the National Academy for State Health Policy states that, "*States may want to require that these*" Enrollee Hold Harmless Clauses "*be part of plan-enrollee contracts in order to better defend them as insurance regulation.*" In other words, the states' own policy manual is telling the Commonwealth of Pennsylvania and the insurance companies that they need to include the Enrollee Hold Harmless Clause in Sandy's insurance plan, rather than a Provider Contract, if they want the Clause to be defensible, (See Exhibit #4). Consequently, there is just no way that the defendants in our litigation could have been unaware of this controlling document and its position on the Enrollee Hold Harmless Clause! The document was written specifically for them! And, given that and the number of times that these defendants repeated the mantra of "*there is nothing in Sandy's Plan that could have possibly barred us from paying for her care,*" the subterfuge can only have been deliberate.

The third response is yet another attempt to deflect our question because the Pennsylvania Code (law) clearly states the Enrollee Hold Harmless Clause is an insolvency provision (See Exhibit #3). --- <u>There is absolutely no mention of balance billing in the regulation</u>. The Blue Cross Blue Shield Association published "Healthcare Coverage Glossary" (http:/www.bcbs.com/coverage/glossary/) provides additional evidence of what can only be seen as the defendants' deliberate misrepresentation of the Clause. The Glossary states: "**hold harmless provision**: *A contract clause which forbids providers from seeking compensation from patients if the health plan fails to compensate the providers because of insolvency ---.*"

In fact, if Pennsylvania had wanted a balance billing provision, they could have simply enacted a prohibition on balance billing. Such provisions are easily written, limited to balance billing, and exist in many states across the country. --- Balance billing being defined as the practice of billing a subscriber for the difference between what a provider has agreed to bill an insurance company and what the provider would "like" to bill for a service rendered to a subscriber. --- However, Pennsylvania, as has every state in the country with the possible exception of Alaska, has chosen to enact the Enrollee Hold Harmless Clause that was written by the National Association of Insurance Commissioners to defend the states as "*zealous guardians of their insurance prerogatives*" in cases of HMO insolvency (An Overview of Bankruptcy & Insurance

28

Insolvency Procedures, Department of Health policy, GWU School of Public Health and Health Services, 2003). In other words, **Pennsylvania, and every other state, have elected to enact the Enrollee Hold Harmless Clause as an absolute ban against providers billing subscribers for *"Covered Services"* in order to defend their ability to regulate health care insurance companies (particularly managed care operations) in instances of insolvency.** However, because Pennsylvania, the other states and the entire insurance industry know that the Enrollee Hold Harmless Clause can't be defended as an insolvency provision, they have chosen to call it a "balance billing provision."--- Far better to describe it as something we would all applaud then to acknowledge the true purpose and draw questions for which there are no defensible answers! --- Interestingly, the states that have enacted a specific ban on balanced billing have enacted additional legislation requiring the Enrollee Hold Harmless Clause.

Returning to the three responses we got to our question of how we could have paid for Sandy's care, I can understand why Sandy's insurance company would attempt to ridicule our question. They were being sued and, as such, had every right to do whatever they could to get the case dismissed. That's our judicial system. However, the State had no such cover. They had a very clear duty to answer our questions fully and accurately. While the insurance companies were within their rights to hide behind the counter intuitive nature of our question, the State had no such right. In fact, one could argue the insurance companies were only parroting the State's misrepresentation of the Enrollee Hold Harmless Clause.

Remember, all we were ever asking in our litigation was for the defendants (Aetna, Blue Cross and the Commonwealth of Pennsylvania) to explain how we could have paid for Sandy's care given the language of the Enrollee Hold Harmless Clause. Yet not one time did they ever directly claim the doctor and the hospitals were free to bill us and accept our money. Not one time did they even attempt to identify a form we could have used, a person we could have contacted to get authorization for a direct payment or anything else we could have done to pay for Sandy's care. Not one time in ten years of litigation and five separate suits. Instead, they steadfastly chose to mislead the court by stressing we were always "free" to pay for a *"Non-Covered Service"* and implying a *"Non-Covered Service"* is anything the insurer refuses to pay for. Both, being statements that are false on their face or, at a minimum, deliberately misleading. See Exhibits 7 & 8 for additional evidence of this deliberate misrepresentation. And please note the underlining in Exhibit 8. The underlining was very carefully done by the author of the letter in what can only be seen as an example of the insurance industry's willingness to deliberately misrepresent the effect of the Enrollee Hold Harmless Clause on subscribers. Representative Art Hershey was one of the most senior members of the Pennsylvania Legislature. So the letter demonstrates not only the insurer's willingness to misrepresent the Clause, but just how brazen and confident they are in this misrepresentation.

I can't leave this letter to Representative Hershey without asking you to please study it carefully. It's an absolutely perfect example of what my family faced throughout our litigation. Not one word in this letter can be individually cited as wrong or actionable. However, the way the words have been strung together and carefully underlined conveys an understanding that is not only misleading and false, but I maintain, deliberately misleading and false. Furthermore, the letter provides us with an example of just how far

up this misrepresentation goes. It's a letter from Office of Legislative Policy for one of the most prominent insurers in the country to one of the most senior members in the Pennsylvania Legislature. Exhibit #7 provides an even longer and more obvious example of this willingness to deliberately mislead subscribers on "*Covered Services*" and their ability to self-pay for necessary health care.

Black's Law Dictionary defines fraud as "*a knowing misrepresentation of the truth or concealment of a material fact to induce another to act to his or her determent.*" And while the states have different approaches to defining actionable fraud, we can pretty much cover the field by citing three primary elements needed to prove actionable fraud. The first element is that the defendant has to have knowingly made a false statement of fact. The second element is that the statement has to have been made with an intent that a party rely on it. And the third element is that the reliance has to be detrimental to the party, i.e., the party suffered quantifiable damage by that reliance. So let's take a close look at whether I am justified in using the term fraud to characterize the actions of the insurance companies and government.

In terms of Element #1, the Pennsylvania Department of Insurance knows full well that the Enrollee Hold Harmless Clause is an insolvency provision to prevent providers from pursuing subscribers under any circumstances, because their own state regulations say exactly that. An insurance company can know no less. Consequently, to stipulate anything else (to maintain that its intent is solely to prevent balance billing) can only be a deliberate attempt to misrepresent and conceal the truth as they know it. --- To knowingly mislead and conceal the fact that by accepting an HMO policy from her employer, Sandy had surrendered her right to pay for her own health care. And if Sandy surrendered that right, so has every subscriber whose policy is subject to an insurance company's Provider Contract and the Enrollee Hold Harmless Clause. Quoting from the Office of the U.S. Attorney General's letter to the White House on this very issue, "*a more difficult issue is raised if an individual willing to forgo reimbursement of the fee is unable to choose his or her own physician*" or hospital.

Element #2, is even easier to prove because the federal ERISA law mandates that all insurers fully disclose the terms and conditions of their Plans to subscribers. Consequently, the insurer has a duty to disclose the truth about the Enrollee Hold Harmless Clause and Provider Contracts. Furthermore, the subscriber has every right to rely on the accuracy of that disclosure. It's literally the law, and the State and the insurance companies have to know this to be the case.

And as for Element #3, quantifiable damage is all too easy to prove. I trust that few would argue that the death of the 14-year-old daughter I described back on page 14 or the death of Sandy wouldn't qualify as sufficient quantifiable damage for actionable fraud.

By misrepresenting and concealing the full effect of the Enrollee Hold Harmless Clause in private Provider Contracts, the states and the insurance industry have subscribers unknowingly surrendering their ability to freely access health care outside the interference of their insurance company and the state. Once again quoting from the ERISA Preemption Manual for State Health Policy Matters published by the National Academy for State Health Policy, "*States may want to require that these*" Enrollee Hold Harmless Clauses "*be part of plan-enrollee contracts in order to better*

defend them as insurance regulation." In other words, the states need to have subscribers knowingly sign off on these restrictions if they want to be able to defend them as appropriate state action. And both the states and the insurance industry know it!

In searching for additional information for this book, I came across an article on www.healthinsurancecoverage.com, entitled "Three Reasons The Enrollee Hold Harmless Provision Is Good To Have In Your Insurance Policy." The reasons they cite are: 1.) It protects policyholders/subscribers in cases of insurer insolvency; 2.) It stops providers from padding bills with extra treatments, and; 3.) It removes the element of money in the doctor-patient relationship.

There just can't be a better example of the fraud I describe above. This insurance industry blog is telling us why we, as subscribers, should demand the Enrollee hold Harmless Clause be included in our health plans. Just what the National Academy for State Health Policy advised in their ERISA Preemption Manual for State Health Policy Matters. However, nowhere in this propaganda-piece do they bother to mention that by having the Enrollee hold Harmless Clause included in your health policy/plan, you are legally agreeing to allow your insurance company to deny you the right to access health care, i.e., to allow your insurer to decide exactly what care you will be <u>allowed</u> to receive regardless of whether you can pay for it yourself. Furthermore, they make no mention of the fact that by removing the element of money from your doctor-patient relationship, you are surrendering the relationship as a matter of law. If you can't pay your doctor, there can't be a contractual relationship and a duty owed. In other words, the removal of money from the doctor-patient relationship frees your doctor to "comply" with the decisions and procedures of your insurance company.

The one area where I do commend the blog for its honesty is where they acknowledge that the reason for the Enrollee Hold Harmless Clause is to protect subscribers in cases of insurer "<u>insolvency</u>." However, even here they attempt to mislead subscribers for the insurance industry's own gain. Because including the Enrollee Hold Harmless Clause in a subscriber's policy/plan does nothing to protect a subscriber from insurer insolvency. The only way the Enrollee Hold Harmless Clause can provide insolvency protection is to have it included in the insurer's Provider Contracts. Just where it is currently. So the authors of the blog aren't promoting your protection against insurer insolvency. They are trying to make the loss of your right to freely access health care <u>defensible</u> in a court of law.

Once again, it just can't be any clearer that the insurance industry and its raft of supporters, including the states, aren't interested in protecting you as a subscriber or your rights under the U. S. Constitution and almost certainly your rights under every state constitution in the country. No, this is about surrendering the rights of the individual in order to strengthen the private health care insurance industry. It's about deliberate misrepresentation and fraud in the pursuit of a stronger bottom line for insurance companies. It's about instituting a private rationing system to reduce the national cost of health care. It's about hiding this egregious affront to our sense of fairness and honest dealings.

As I stated earlier, if the Enrollee Hold Harmless Clause was solely intended to prevent balanced billing, as the states maintain, they could simply add language that would allow a subscriber to elect to pay whenever their insurance company refuses to pay. But they

don't, and there is a very good reason why. If the states were to allow a subscriber to elect to pay for a Covered Service, then the agreement that each of us sign when we are admitted to a hospital would completely nullify the Enrollee Hold Harmless Clause. You know the one, the clause that has us agreeing to accept responsibility for whatever our insurance company fails to pay. In short, the form that we all sign prior to receiving care would eliminate the state's insolvency provision and once again threaten the states' right to regulate health insurance.

A perfect example of this can be found in our dealings with the Leader of the Pennsylvania State Senate, Senator Dominic Pileggi. I had contacted the Senator hoping to get his help with our case and the issue we were trying to raise. In responding, the Senator made the mistake of believing the intent of the Clause was to prevent balance billing and drafted legislation (Senate Bill No 1184 of Session 2006) that would have limited the reach of the Enrollee Hold Harmless Clause and allow subscribers to *"enter into an agreement with the provider to obtain the services at the covered individual's own expense"*. Needless to say, the measure never came up for a vote and was effectively buried before the ink was dry. The Senator also dropped out of sight as far as the Lobbs and the issue were concerned. He was just no longer available to us!

This was the Republican leader of the Pennsylvania Senate, a lawyer AND the <u>brother of Sandy's doctor</u>. So there can be no question that he came to understand this issue fully. I spoke with him too many times, and I'm sure he spoke with his sister, who was adamant about the injustice of the Enrollee Hold Harmless Clause. He simply ran into the true intent of the Clause, along with its politics, and was forced to back away. I mention him here not to be critical, but to provide an example of just how powerful the forces are that are behind this fraud on the American people. --- A fraud that goes all the way to the top of the Republican Party and their adopted Ryan Budget.

However, just so I am not seen as solely dumping on the Republican Party, the Democratic Party can be shown to have been responsible for attempting to establish a provision in federal law that would have placed the same restriction on Medicare beneficiaries that the Enrollee Hold Harmless Clause places on subscribers of private insurance.

Ever since the enactment of Medicare in 1965, there have been concerns that the program would lead to rationing and the denial of a beneficiary's right to pay for care outside the Medicare system. For those interested in a detailed analysis of those concerns and issues, there is an excellent paper available through the Cato Institute, dated October 15, 2007, entitled "The Freedom to Spend Your Own Money on Medical Care" by Kent Masterson Brown. However, for the purposes of this book, we will only cover the highlights as they apply to the fraud surrounding the Enrollee Hold Harmless Clause.

In 1997, in what was clearly a Democratic push to restrict the ability of Medicare beneficiaries to pay for services outside the Medicare system, the Clinton administration negotiated what became known as Section 4507 of the Balanced Budget Act of 1997. Under that Section, if a physician were to provide even a single Medicare-covered service to a single self-paying Medicare beneficiary, that physician would have been completely barred from treating Medicare patients for a period of two years.

The practical effect of this was that Medicare beneficiaries would only be able to self-pay doctors who had chosen to opt out of Medicare entirely, an essentially impossible financial decision for physicians given the volume of Medicare patients in their practices. In essence, Section 4507 provided the same restrictions on beneficiaries self-paying for care in the Medicare system that the Enrollee Hold Harmless Clause imposes on subscribers with private insurance. Unfortunately for the Clinton Administration and the Democrats, Section 4507 was both visible and highly controversial. The result was that the United Seniors Association, with a long list of supporting parties, challenged the constitutionality of Section 4507 in federal court. That case is United Seniors Association et al. v. Shalala.

The end result of this case was that the Clinton Administration and its Health and Human Services Secretary (Donna Shalala) were so intimidated by the specter of having to defend their restrictions on beneficiaries self-paying for necessary health care that they completely rewrote the provision and retreated from the issue. They ran from the fight. In other words, they assured the court that they (the federal government) accepted a beneficiary's right to self-pay for care that was not approved or supplied by Medicare.

The relevance of this case to the Enrollee Hold Harmless Clause and fraud is that the insurance industry and state governments are fully aware of the decision in United Seniors Association et al. v. Shalala. Consequently, they know that if forced to defend their carefully constructed and hidden Enrollee Hold Harmless Clause, they will lose the fight. And, given the fact that the Enrollee Hold Harmless Clause is the very foundation upon which the insurance industry has built its world and profits, can any of us be surprised at what I am characterizing as a clear and deliberate fraud aimed at hiding the issue?

V.   How We Got Here (History of the Enrollee Hold Harmless Clause)

In the late 1980s, the exploding growth of HMOs overheated in a number of unsettling HMO insolvencies. Even more unsettling was that in the largest of these insolvencies, Maxicare HMOs, the HMO was granted relief under Chapter 11 of the Federal Bankruptcy Code. This marked a significant departure from what had been the accepted practice and the prevailing view of applicable law, because the Federal Bankruptcy Code specifically excludes a "domestic insurance company" from being granted such protection. An exception in the law aimed specifically at recognizing the authority of the states to regulate insurance.

In the Maxicare case, the court ruled that, while an HMO has many of the same features as an indemnity insurer ("domestic insurance company"), there are certain distinguishing characteristics that make HMOs quite different. In other words, the court held that a HMO is not a "domestic insurance company" and therefore not barred from the protections available under the federal bankruptcy statutes, --- protections that move an insolvent HMO out from under the control of the state and its established authority to regulate insurance.

The significance of this threat to what the states considered their private turf can't be overstated. For while the federal court's ruling in Maxicare focused on HMOs, it really threatened to include all managed care organizations (MCOs). This concept of "managed care" covered an enormous variety of insurance models and the overwhelming bulk of the nation's health care insurance companies. In short, the Maxicare ruling threatened to effectively eliminate the authority of the

states to regulate health care insurance as they had known it. From 1970 to 1999, HMO enrollment alone exploded from 3 million to more than 80 million subscribers as Conservatives pushed to make HMOs the primary vehicle for controlling the nation's runaway cost of health care.

The murkiness of this jurisdictional dispute between the states and the federal courts was further exacerbated by the irony that MCOs were actively pressing the courts to view them as health care companies in order to qualify for federal bankruptcy protection while pressing these very same courts to view them as domestic insurance companies when it came to charges of medical malpractice. In other words, HMOs and all other forms of managed care wanted to have it both ways. On one hand, they were arguing that they should not be viewed as insurance companies for the purpose of bankruptcy (the Maxicare ruling). On the other hand, they were just as active in arguing that they should be viewed as insurance companies in all matters of medical malpractice so that they could escape liability for denying care.

Once again, for those who wish to explore the details of the controversy created by the "Maxicare HMOs" decision, those details can be readily found in a host of articles, papers, court records and books available over the internet. However, for our purpose, we really only need to understand the scope of the conflict that was created.

The regulation of insurance had long been viewed as the exclusive authority of the states, a position well supported in rulings by the U. S. Supreme Court. However, the ruling in Maxicare HMOs called all that into question. HMOs were becoming the predominant form of health care insurance. Hence, if the states couldn't regulate HMOs and the other forms of managed care, they would lose much of their authority to regulate health care insurance.

As anyone who has followed the courts knows, resolving an issue this complex and fundamental to the separation of powers is never quick, and rarely decisive. As a result, parties usually look for more readily available solutions in such disputes. And so was the case here. The states were not about to surrender their power to regulate insurance to the federal courts. State regulators had overseen HMOs from the moment of their creation and were not about to have their authority yanked out from under them the moment an HMO was threatened with insolvency.

While this dispute could well be characterized as a turf war, there was an even greater underlying issue. To the states' credit, they and their laws were focused on protecting the rights of subscribers over the rights of an HMO and its network of providers. The Federal Bankruptcy Code clearly bars any such preferential treatment. In fact, the federal court's ruling in "Maxicare HMOs" described the states' efforts to protect subscribers as "*an anathema to the basic tenant of federal bankruptcy law.*" In short, the states stood in united opposition to both the federal court's ruling on the appropriate forum for HMO insolvencies and its rejection of state efforts to protect subscribers.

The answer for the states was not only readily available, but also quite simple. The National Association of Insurance Commissioners (NAIC) published the HMO Model Act to guide states in developing a unified response to the regulatory issues HMOs were creating in the market and allow the states to retain their regulatory authority. More specifically, the Act contained an insolvency provision called the Enrollee Hold Harmless Clause that the states were to add to their regulations and laws. By simply adopting this provision of the NAIC's HMO Model Act, a state could guarantee the protection they sought for subscribers in instances of HMO insolvency and essentially eliminate any justification for federal bankruptcy proceedings. Even more

important, by requiring that the Enrollee Hold Harmless Clause be included in the private Provider Contracts that HMOs must have with their providers, the states eliminate even the ability of the federal courts to draw subscribers into a federal bankruptcy proceeding. Consequently, even if the states were to lose their turf war with the federal courts, they would insure subscribers remained protected and outside the reach of federal bankruptcy. In effect, by requiring the Enrollee Hold Harmless Clause be included in all Provider Contracts, the states isolated subscribers from federal bankruptcy, facilitated state transfer of subscribers to another HMO and undercut the federal court's justification for federal bankruptcy proceedings.

While I have spoken as though all 50 states acted as one, they obviously did not. However, between 1989 and the present, every state in the nation, with the possible exception of Alaska, has adopted the Enrollee Hold Harmless Clause as drafted by the NAIC (a published conclusion of the Maryland Attorney General). And while I make no claim that this, on its own, accounted for the states winning their turf war with the federal courts, the question of the appropriate forum for HMO insolvency proceedings appears both resolved in the favor of the states and firmly in the past.

In summary, by adopting the National Association of Insurance Commissioners' insolvency provision, the Enrollee Hold Harmless Clause, the states have been able to retain their broad authority to regulate health care insurance by preventing subscribers from becoming parties to federal bankruptcy proceedings. Unfortunately for you, me, Sandy and all other subscribers, the states' adoption of the Enrollee Hold Harmless Clause has done a great deal more.

VI. Why Prevent A Subscriber From Paying for Health Care?

A. The Insurance Industry's Reason

The question of "why" is one we heard repeatedly throughout our search for an attorney and the litigation process. It's a question that we, quite honestly, completely mishandled. I was so blinded by my anger over the loss of Sandy and our inability to pay for her care that I couldn't see anything but a single out-of-control insurance company denying care for a better bottom line. In fact, it wasn't until very late in the litigation that I was able to step back far enough to recognize just how little sense this explanation made. Allowing a subscriber to pay for his or her own health care would have exactly the same effect on an insurer's bottom line as denying care. In short, the answer I had jumped to so quickly wasn't credible and the attorneys for Sandy's insurer were quick to point it out. How could allowing a subscriber to pay for their own health care represent any skin off the nose of an insurance company? --- So, as I was forced to do, let's step back and take a closer look.

First of all, who hasn't heard that the rising cost of health care isn't sustainable? It's cited as one of the country's largest problems. In fact, the Ryan Budget Proposal for the Republican Party identifies this as one of its primary drivers. However, Congressman Ryan's proposal is just another in literally years of attempts to bring the cost of health care under control, attempts that led to the explosive rise of the HMO as a primary tool for reigning in the cost of health care.

Initially developed in the 1930's, HMOs grew slowly for the next few decades. However, in the 1970's, powerful conservative voices began to embrace the HMO as an alternative

to socialized medicine and President Nixon boosted the HMO into prominence by signing the HMO Act of 1973. By the late 1970's, the stock market was fully on board and HMOs were rapidly becoming for-profit businesses. However, it was the country's broad recognition of the need to control the cost of health care in the 1980's through to the present that can be best cited for the growth of HMOs and managed care in general. Because of their unique ability to negotiate lower costs from doctors, hospitals and other health care providers, these new forms of insurance were viewed as offering a free-market solution to the problem. Consequently, federal and state governments increasingly threw their support behind the growth of these new forms of insurance.

As with any negotiations, the ability of HMOs to successfully negotiate lower costs depended largely on being able to get the participating parties to the table. However, so long as doctors and hospitals were free to practice outside HMO networks, the providers could ignore both the HMOs and the opportunity these negotiations offered for lowering the cost of health care. Enter, once again, the NAIC and their HMO Model Act, which encouraged the states to require that every doctor and hospital that participates with an HMO have a Provider Contract. Or, stated another way, every doctor and hospital that wishes to participate with an HMO must come to the table and negotiate a formal Provider Contract with that HMO. Problem solved. The states accepted the recommendations of the NAIC and given the volume of business that HMO patients represented to providers, the doctors and hospitals across the country simply could not refuse to come to the table. They couldn't afford to lose the business.

With doctors and hospitals effectively forced to negotiate with the HMOs, the promised power of the HMOs to negotiate lower costs became a reality. However, to assume that doctors and hospitals were given the freedom to negotiate terms and conditions in these Provider Contracts would be a mistake. The states not only required the completion of these Contracts, they mandated the inclusion of specific provisions and language, including the Enrollee Hold Harmless Clause, and insisted the Contracts be reviewed and approved by the state. The result has been that the doctors and hospitals have been handed essentially completed agreements and given little choice but to sign. The only portion open for negotiation has been an attachment at the back of the Contract that establishes the rates a provider agrees to use for billing Covered Services. And even here, I doubt there are many doctors or hospitals that would see these negotiations on billing rates as fair and open. By their very design, HMOs were to have a unique ability to force providers to accept lower rates.

By being able to force doctors and hospitals to sign what are clearly very one-sided Provider Contracts, everyone but the providers got what they were seeking from HMOs and managed care. As I described above, the states absolutely had to have the insolvency protection that the Enrollee Hold Harmless Clause provides. Insurers, on the other hand, had to have complete control over what doctors could prescribe and hospitals could render a subscriber in order to deliver an acceptable bottom line. And lastly, state and federal government had to see a reduction in the cost of health care.

The significance of all this is that the Provider Contract became the foundation stone upon which HMOs and the other forms of managed care have built their dominance in the market as well as the focal point for one of the nation's most important efforts to reduce the runaway cost of health care. These Provider Contracts are literally the heart of

the business model upon which the insurance industry depends for its power and profits. In addition, these Contracts are directly responsible for delivering the only measurable success in the nation's efforts to rein in the rapidly escalating cost of health care. In other words, these Provider Contracts are the foundation upon which the majority of this nation's private health care system has been built.

The key to the success of the HMOs and the other forms of managed care has very clearly been their ability to not only control the cost of the care being delivered, but the nature of that care as well. For, while having the power to negotiate lower rates might seem to be an answer in itself, it's a temporary answer at best. All products and services represent a cost to a provider beyond which no amount of negotiating can hope to succeed in lowering the billing rate a provider can charge an insurer. In essence, negotiations on billing rates can only yield diminishing returns. Once a provider's margin of profit is cut to the bone, the only future savings available through negotiations are those that can be obtained through improvements in efficiency. --- And so we come to the denial of care.

The single most important factor in determining the efficiency of the care delivered to a subscriber is the nature and amount of the care prescribed by the doctor. Eliminate a test, simplify a treatment, substitute an alternative cheaper drug or reduce the number of days a patient remains in the hospital and you have an immediate improvement in efficiency. It's simple math. And given the maturity of the HMOs and managed care, it's the math driving their negotiations with providers. It's the only math capable of delivering an acceptable bottom line and acceptable growth for the insurance industry; and, delivering a solution for the nation's unsustainable cost of health care, --- both leveraged on HMOs' (managed care's) ability to deny care.

But what does this have to do with a need to deny subscribers the ability to pay for their own care or our ability to pay for the care prescribed for Sandy? The answer is quite simple. If you refer back to the section in this book entitled "The Heart of The Fraud", you will see that Enrollee Hold Harmless Clause can only be interpreted as barring any and all such payments for *"Covered Services."* *"Covered Services"* being defined in law and contract as the services contained in the benefit package of a subscriber's Plan regardless of whether the insurer elects to approve and pay for the service in a particular instance. It's both the law and the protection the states have instituted against the federal courts usurping their right to regulate HMOs in cases of insolvency.

So we arrive at the answer for why the insurance industry would deny subscribers the ability to self-pay for their own health care. The truth is that an insurer doesn't have the authority to allow a subscriber to self-pay for a *"Covered Service."* They literally lack any and all authority to ignore the Enrollee Hold Harmless Clause's absolute bar on subscriber's paying for a *"Covered Service."* Moreover, were they to ignore the bar, they would be undercutting the very core of their Provider Contracts, their business model, their ability to negotiate with providers and the very foundation for their power in the market. In essence, the insurance industry can't allow subscribers to pay for their own health care without knowingly violating the law and severely damaging themselves in the market.

Once again, why would an insurance company deny their subscribers the right to pay for their own health care? Because it's a key element in a carefully constructed scheme that neither the insurance industry nor state governments want called into question or disclosed to the public. A scheme literally built on the backs of Provider Contracts that provide the engine for managed care's dominance in this country's health care system. Dominance that is not only allowed, but actively supported at all levels of state and federal government. And, yes we are talking countless billions of dollars set against the right of an individual subscriber to pay for his or her own health care.

Now this is where someone always steps forward to claim they know of a HMO subscriber who was allowed to pay for their own health care; as if this somehow sets aside state law and the language contained in Provider Contracts. My answer is always the same. I explain that I just happen to know an individual who drove through a red-light and wasn't ticked. In fact, I have done it myself. However, to the best of my knowledge, running a red-light is still against the law.

Yes, there are certainly instances where providers have improperly billed subscribers and the subscribers have self-paid for the care they received. So long as no one complains to the state department of insurance about balanced billing or the insurer is ignorant of the issue or willing to turn a blind eye, who is going to step in and draw attention to the Enrollee old Harmless Clause. However, make the situation one in which the insurer has refused to pre-certify an expensive course of treatment and you can bet the insurer will be taking steps to enforce the terms of their Provider Contract. After all, insurers don't move against subscribers to restrict access to health care. They sanction the provider; sanctions that can easily drive a provider into bankruptcy. It's the threat of these devastating sanctions that allows insurers to enforce their bar against subscribers self-paying for care, not some state enforcement action. Go back to page 14 and read the testimony of Jeffrey A. Thomas on this very issue.

Summarizing why the insurance industry would deny you the right to pay for your own health care:

1) HMOs are required to have a state approved Provider Contract with every doctor, hospital and other service provider in their network of approved providers.

2) Each of these Provider Contracts must include the Enrollee Hold Harmless Clause that forces providers to surrender any and all right to bill subscribers for *"Covered Services"* and voids any agreement subscribers think they have with their doctor or hospital.

3) *"Covered Services"* are defined in law and Provider Contracts as the services contained in the benefit package of a subscriber's Plan regardless of whether the insurer elects to approve and pay for the service in a particular instance.

4) Insurers add provisions to their Provider Contracts that further restrict the ability of providers to bill subscribers and enhance the ability of insurers to override the decisions of a subscriber's doctor.

5) Insurers broaden the applicability of Provider Contracts by having them apply to all products under their corporate name and all other affiliated business entities.

6) Insurers include language that requires doctors and hospitals to support and comply with an insurer's decisions, policies and practices.

7) Insurers further require doctors and hospitals to provide necessary and appropriate care <u>regardless</u> of whether the insurer is willing to approve and pay for the care.

8) Insurers declare their state approved Provider Contracts (public documents) to be proprietary business information that cannot be disclosed.

9) **And lastly, allowing a provider to bill a subscriber in violation of their Provider Contract and, more specifically the Enrollee Hold Harmless Clause, would breach the Agreement and establish a precedent that would invite litigation that could easily result in the collapse of the entire HMO business model.**

Note: I don't even have to defend Point #9 because it's the written opinion of the insurance industry and government.

Quoting from the ERISA Preemption Manual for State Health Policy Matters published by the National Academy for State Health Policy, "*States may want to require that these*" Enrollee Hold Harmless Clauses "*be part of plan-enrollee contracts in order to better defend them as insurance regulation.*" The context here is that states need to recognize that if their current use of the Enrollee Hold Harmless Clause is challenged in federal court, it is likely to be held to be a violation of ERISA, federal law and the U. S. Constitution. A more defensible position would be to include the Enrollee Hold Harmless Clause in a subscriber's plan where it can be accepted and signed by the subscriber.

And, quoting from a letter to the White House from the Department of Justice, "*legislation that restricts individual's ability to select their own physicians will invite attack on the grounds that it interferes with a constitutional right of privacy.*" --- "*But a more difficult issue is raised if an individual willing to forgo reimbursement of the fee is unable to choose his or her own physician.*" The context here is to answer the White House's questions, and I quote ("*concerning the possible constitutionality of different options concerning regulation and delivery of health care services*").

B. Your Insurance Company's Additional Reason

Under the laws of every state, only a properly licensed physician can prescribe necessary or appropriate health care. These same laws make it crystal clear that hospitals can only supply care that has been properly prescribed and must supply that care so long as payment is available.

Now consider what would have happened if we had been allowed to pay for Sandy's care and then sued to recover the cost. The insurance company would be on record having refused to approve the care on the grounds that it was not "medically necessary or appropriate". However, by providing the care we sought for Sandy, the doctor and hospital would have demonstrated the care she received <u>was</u> "medically necessary and appropriate." Under state law, the care they delivered could be nothing less. The only alternative would be if one or both had violated the law, in which case, one or both would be open to charges of malpractice, incompetence and fraud. Not a likely situation and certainly not something they are going to admit.

Consequently, if we, or any other subscriber, sued their insurance company to recover the cost of care they had received and paid for, so long as it was an available benefit (a "*Covered Service*") and the insurer had denied coverage on the basis that the care was not "medically necessary or appropriate," the insurer would be in a very deep hole. They would be faced with a significant lawsuit with essentially no defense. The actions of the doctor and the hospital would provide clear proof that the care was "medically necessary and appropriate" under law. In addition, the subscriber's plan would show that the insurer promising to provide the care so long as it was "medically necessary or appropriate." And, were the insurer to raise elements of its Provider Contract and the Enrollee Hold Harmless Clause in its defense, it would likely do very little to reduce the insurer's liability while opening the entire matter of their Provider contracts and Enrollee Hold Harmless Clause to review and scrutiny. --- A completely no-win situation for the insurer, and for the state as well.

On the other hand, if the subscriber never gets the care, the insurer has solid proof that the care was not "medically necessary or appropriate," because, doctors and hospitals, must provide that care whenever it is required ("medically necessary or appropriate"). And since the care was not provided, the insurer has very solid prima-facie evidence the care was not needed and therefore cannot qualify for coverage. Or stated slightly differently, if the care was never needed, there can have been no damage. No denied "necessary and appropriate" care or damage, no basis for suit. --- Or once again, no harm, no foul.

The bottom line is that your insurance company has every reason to insure that you, or any other subscriber, are never allowed to pay for care that is an available benefit, but the insurer has denied coverage because they alone have determined the care is not "medically necessary and/or appropriate." They absolutely must retain what amounts to an essentially unrestricted ability to deny coverage and care in order to grow their profits and bonuses.

In testimony before Congress, Wendell Potter, a former head of corporate communications for CIGNA (one of the largest health care insurers in the country), stated that the average family doesn't understand how much the demands of Wall Street dictate whether a subscriber will be afforded coverage. He went on to say that the top priority of for-profit insurers is to "*drive up the value of their stock.*" And, one of the most important factors in accomplishing this is to drive down the company's "*benefit ratio*," (the ratio between what an insurer actually pays out in claims and what it has left over for overhead and profit). He testified that he had seen an insurer's stock price fall twenty percent in a single day for an increase in their benefit ratio of just 77.9% to 79.4% in a year. He further testified that a study conducted by PricewaterhouseCoopers revealed just how successful insurers have been in exploiting this "benefit ratio" to improve their profitability. From 1998 to 2008, the insurance industry saw this critical ratio fall from 85.3% to 81.6%. A result that can only have come from an increase in the industry's denial of coverage and care.

Quoting Mr. Potter, "*Claims denials are probably the most effective way the industry has to manage medical expenses*", (Center for American Progress article entitled "Insurer's Black Box").

C. Government's Reason

While we all think of our health care insurance as "our own" personal policy, nothing could be further from the truth for most Americans. The vast majority of us receive our health insurance through our employer as part of an employee benefit package. Furthermore, most of this insurance is in the form of an HMO Plan or some other form of managed care insurance. In essence, it isn't insurance as we have historically defined it and we certainly do not own it.

While most of us have never given any serious thought to why we are called "subscribers", "enrollees" or "members" instead of policyholders, it's really something we need to understand. Rather than having a direct contractual relationship with an insurance company, as you do with your homeowner's policy, we are simply being granted participation in our employer's health "Plan". Consequently, there is no direct contractual obligation owed to a subscriber (you) by the Plan's insurance company.

Why is this important? Well, as I have shown above, by making you a subscriber/enrollee/member in your employer's Plan, your employer is effectively surrendering your right to access health care outside the Plan. But, by what authority, and where is your informed consent? Not only that, but your employer is doing it because your state government is requiring it. Boy oh boy, if there was ever a case for the 14th Amendment of the U. S. Constitution and due process, this has to be it.

My point is that both the state and federal governments are fully aware of the issue. See the quotes from ERISA Preemption Manual for State Health Policy Matters (Exhibit #4) and the Letter to the White House from the Department of Justice in Section (A). However, given that the loss of your right to access health care outside your employer's Plan is at the very heart of the managed care business model, just how ready do you think government is to opening this issue up to review by the public and the courts? --- We are talking about the potential collapse of the entire health insurance industry as we know it.

If insurers can't restrict subscribers' access to care, they can't control their providers and they can't control the cost of care. And if they can't control the cost of care, they literally don't bring any value to the market and would be headed for certain extinction.

We are talking about billions of dollars in cost, monumental changes to state and federal law and a potential for class action suits that should put a gleam in the eye of every aspiring litigator in the country. Countless people have died because employers have improperly surrendered their employees' right to access health care outside their employer's Plan. Again, I am not a lawyer, but employers have a responsibility and a duty under law to, at a minimum, disclose the terms of their Plans. It's a responsibility and duty that they have clearly breached and continue to breach. The irony is that employers would be first in line for suits in this area while the truly responsible parties (the insurance companies) would be standing well in the background claiming "no harm, no foul".

Simply put, the growth of HMOs and managed care has been driven by the Conservatives' pursuit of an alternative to socialized medicine and the nation's very real need to reduce the cost of health care. Reductions that can be shown to have been

41

produced by managed care. Now add to this mix the states' use of the Enrollee Hold Harmless Clause to defend their authority to regulate health insurance and do you really have to ask why government wouldn't want this carefully constructed world (HMOs and other forms of managed care financed by employers) to implode? --- I hope not!!!

VII. How They Hide It from You

To keep something this large a secret, you have to do more than just try to hide the documents. After all, the Enrollee Hold Harmless Clause is readily available in the regulations and the laws of essentially every state in the country. People are going to see it. So, the insurance industry and government have had to find a way to hide it in plain sight. Fortunately for them, all they had to do was tweak the stated purpose of the Clause. The states could simply change their description of the Enrollee Hold Harmless Clause from an insolvency provision with an absolute bar against subscribers paying for their own health care to a balanced billing provision enacted to protect subscribers from unfair billing practices. And while the wording of the Clause would appear to make this "tweaking" rather simple, we need to take a closer look if we want to understand just how clever these folks have been.

To begin with, the wording in the Clause makes it very clear that it *"shall be construed to be for the benefit of the Subscriber."* Nowhere in the Clause, or anywhere else that I have ever been able to find, is there even a hint of exactly what this benefit is supposed to be. It's simply left to the imagination of the reader, and, as I will explain below, the states. What is clear is that if you are a state regulator or the employee of an insurance company, you must represent the Clause as purely for the benefit of subscribers.

Unfortunately for the states and the insurance industry, if you read the Pennsylvania Code (**§301.121. Protections Against Insolvency**), any number of other references I have cited throughout the book, and countless other references that are readily available, it simply can't be more clear than that the Enrollee Hold Harmless Clause is, and was specifically written as, an insolvency provision with an absolute bar against subscribers self-paying for "Covered Services". However, if you call the Pennsylvania Department of Health or Insurance, I can guarantee you will be told *"the intent of the Enrollee Hold Harmless Clause is to prevent providers from Balance Billing subscribers."* I've heard it all too many times! --- So how can a state be this bold in misrepresenting its own law? How can a state refuse to address the actual language and the designed intent of the Enrollee Hold Harmless Clause? How can states and the insurance industry refuse to acknowledge the absolute bar against self-payment contained in the Clause?

What makes all the obfuscation and misrepresentation possible for the states and the insurance industry (to literally hide the Clause in plain sight) is a longstanding holding of the U. S. Supreme Court. Under *Chevron U.S.A. Inc. v. National Resources Defense Council, Inc.*, if a statute is ambiguous we must defer to an agency's reasonable interpretation of its terms. 467 U.S. 837,842-45 (1984); *see United States v. Haggar Apparel Co.*, 119 S. Ct. 1395 (1999). *This is so regardless whether there may be other reasonable, or even more reasonable interpretations.* See Serono Labs., Inc. v. Shalala, 158 F.3d 1313, 1321 (D.C. Cir. 1998).

In essence, the Supreme Court has empowered the states to describe the Enrollee Hold Harmless Clause as they see fit. So if they choose to describe it in the laudable terms of a balance billing provision for the benefit of subscribers, they are fully within their rights to do so. And, since the

states have adopted this description, the insurance industry is fully within their rights to sing the same song. Each insurance company secure in the knowledge that they are simply following pronouncements of the state and rulings of the U. S. Supreme Court. --- Deliberate misrepresentation, Yes! But, a clear and chargeable lie, --- No!

It's the perfect sham. The states have no need to enforce the Enrollee Hold Harmless Clause as an insolvency provision because once it's in an insurer's private Provider Contract it automatically takes on the role of an insolvency provision under well-established contract law. Consequently, the states are free to enforce the Clause solely as a balance billing provision knowing full well that under contract law the Clause can only be interpreted as an absolute bar against billing subscribers. The operative word here being "enforce." On one hand, the states have to enforce a ban on balance billing because subscribers (voters) have shown they won't tolerate such unfair billing practices. On the other hand, there is no need for the states to enforce the clause as an insolvency provision because it's the doctor's and the hospital's burden to show they have a right to bill subscribers in an insolvency proceeding. And given the clear and unambiguous language of the Clause, there is no way that doctors and hospitals can ever meet that burden. By requiring what the states describe as a balance billing provision be included in every Provider Contract, the states guarantee that contracted doctors and hospitals can never demonstrate a right to bill subscribers in all cases of insurer insolvency or for any other reason involving "*Covered Services.*"

However, probably the greatest reason why questions around the Enrollee Hold Harmless Clause never surface is that the entire matter is so counterintuitive. Who in their right mind would ever question his or her right or ability to pay for their own health care? Yet, even in this choice of words I have raised a point that no one would ever think to question. Reasonable people would naturally assume the right to pay and the ability to pay are one and the same. Unfortunately, it just isn't true here. The legal minds responsible for creating this masterful piece of deception have made the right to pay separate and distinct from one's ability to pay. Consequently, the state and your insurance company are completely free to assure you that your "right" to pay for health care is completely unaffected by their Provider Contracts and the Enrollee Hold Harmless Clause, all the while knowing that these very same agreements and provisions bar your "ability" to pay for necessary and appropriate health care.

It took us years to understand that the "right" to pay is different from an "ability" to pay when it comes to health insurance and interpreting the Enrollee Hold Harmless Clause. In our simple minds, the act of paying requires two things: 1.) There has to be an offer to pay from a buyer; and, 2.) The seller has to accept the payment. I'm absolutely certain I would have no trouble getting agreement on this simple definition from my local bank. Unfortunately, I had no such luck with the various courts hearing our litigation. Sandy's insurer literally beat us to death on this simple but highly effective differentiation. It allowed them to indignantly argue that there was clearly nothing in Sandy's plan that could have possibly altered our "right" to pay for the care she needed.

The icing on the cake is that very few subscribers ever attempt to pay for care. Typically, they can't afford to pay, so the issue of the Enrollee Hold Harmless Clause never surfaces. And if it somehow does surface, the state's assurance that the Clause is solely intended to prevent balance billing and subscribers are completely free to pay for all non-covered services directs the subscriber into the insurance industry's maze of appeals and process. An intentional Gordian knot of circuitous frustration!

Just look at our case for example. I've already acknowledged that it took me years of continuous litigation to recognize that the problem we faced wasn't an out-of-control insurance company perverting the well-intended laws and regulations of the state. Add in the state's and the insurance industry's misleading use of critical definitions (**Please** read section XI. Definitions You Need to Win) and my use of the term "Gordian knot" simply can't be an overstatement! And this doesn't begin to take into account all the misleading information the hospital will be feeding a subscriber being denied coverage and care. Hospitals know they are first in line for a lawsuit and will be doing everything possible to convince a subscriber that what is being done is completely reasonable given the limits of the subscriber's coverage.

I can say this with great confidence because I am known within the world of health care reform as *"the one who tried to pay for his own health care."* Not one of many or one of a few, but the one. In fact, if you go to Google you will find elements of our case under any number of searches. You won't find any mention of a similar case or litigation, at least as far as I have ever been able to find. It seems that there has just never been a subscriber as hard headed and determined as the Lobbs.

The bottom line is that we really have to give the states and the insurance industry some well-earned credit. These are very smart people. They have developed a scheme where they can literally lie to a subscriber's face and be completely credible under law; to deny patients their constitutional right of access to necessary health care without ever having to acknowledge doing it or revealing how it was done; to hide this absolute infringement of our most basic freedoms in plain sight and literally condemn an individual to death for a stronger bottom line and then walk away untouched. As I said, these are extremely smart people!

VIII. Your Doctor's Conundrum & the Solution You Can Provide

I have spent the earlier portions of this book lumping doctors and hospitals together because they sign the same Provider Contracts with the same insurance companies. So, both can be said to be subject to the very same hidden terms and conditions that restrict a subscriber's access to health care. However, if we look more closely at these two classes of providers, there are some very significant differences.

The most obvious differences are size and structure. Hospitals are typically large corporate organizations with all the characteristics and trappings of any modern U. S. business. They have CEOs, CFOs and boards of directors, as well as directors of this and directors of that. They also have large multi-level staffs with a team of attorneys on retainer and probably at least one on staff. In short, hospitals are organizations that you and I can no more have a personal relationship with than we can with General Electric or IBM. They are simply large corporate entities focused on delivering products and services to customers (patients, in this case) for an acceptable bottom line.

Doctors, on the other hand, are different. They are individuals. In fact, the law requires that they practice as individuals. While we all know of a clinic or medical office with more than one doctor, these doctors are merely sharing the administrative costs for their various individual practices. Doctors have to be licensed and only a qualified individual can be granted a license to practice. So while a personal relationship is completely incompatible with the size and structure

of a hospital, it's not only possible with a doctor, it's the norm. Who among us doesn't have a personal physician or family doctor? It's one of the first questions all of us answer when we fill out those all too many questionnaires on our health history. And, while I can't speak for the rest of you, I certainly haven't ever seen a line requesting the name of my personal or family hospital on one of those questionnaires.

Simply put, most of us not only know our doctor, but have a long standing relationship with him or her that is both personal and intimate. It's a relationship that can be placed on a par with your priest, minister or rabbi. It's a relationship born out of your doctor's decision to serve, and a commitment to the Hippocratic Oath. It's a relationship that not only forces the doctor to stand responsible for literally your life in the eyes of you and your family, but just importantly, the law and the courts. So, while a hospital can be no more than a corporation that provides subscribers with products and services, your doctor is essentially a member of your extended family.

The doctor's conundrum, then is, given the constraints of the insurer's Provider Contract with its Enrollee Hold harmless Clause, how can he or she faithfully fulfill the duty owed to you by relationship, profession, oath and the law? How can he or she bend to the whims of an insurance company when duty demands the doctor prescribe and certify care the insurer refuses to approve? How can the doctor certify care that he or she believes is inadequate simply because the insurer, in violation of the law, has usurped the doctor's authority to prescribe necessary and appropriate care? ---- Every doctor's daily conundrum!

Fortunately, each of us, as subscribers to an insurance company's managed care plan, hold the answer to our doctor's conundrum. For while the last thing insurers, government, and even hospitals, want us to know is that each of us have the right to demand that our doctor's initial prescription of needed care is a "certification" of necessary and appropriate care. In essence, we have the right, under law, to insist that the hospital honor our doctor's prescription of needed care separate from any intervention by an insurance company. Remember, your doctor's primary obligation is to serve you and your specific needs. In fact, even your doctor's Provider Contract will almost certainly make this abundantly clear so the insurer can avoid any accountability for what ends up being prescribed. The insurer is simply using the threat of nonpayment to the hospital as a cudgel to force the hospital to push back against the doctor when an insurer decides to deny coverage (payment) for an available benefit. Remember, your doctor is not only duty-bound to provide the care you need, but is likely to have very few dollars at risk on his determination of necessary and appropriate care. By contrast, the hospital will be facing tens of thousands of dollars in potentially unpaid costs if they provide the care your doctor is prescribing and the insurer is refusing to cover. Consequently, the entire issue is one of cost not care. Your doctor wants to provide the care you need. On the other hand, the hospital will be doing everything possible to avoid getting stuck with the bill.

Fortunately for you and your doctor, hospitals are required to honor your doctor's decisions on necessary and appropriate health care as a matter of law. The only caveat is that hospitals, outside of emergency services, are not required to provide that care free of charge. It has been well held that they aren't charitable institutions and have every right to demand payment for the services they provide. However, all you have to do to bring them under the law is to insist on self-paying for the care your doctor is prescribing, --- assuming, of course, that the care is an available benefit under your insurer's plan. After all, it isn't your or your doctor's fault that the

hospital has voluntarily surrendered the right to bill you or collect your money. They just have to honor your offer to pay and provide the care your doctor is prescribing. It's the law, and almost certainly a requirement of their license to operate.

Once again, per the terms of their Provider Contract with its Enrollee Hold Harmless Clause the hospital has voluntarily agreed *"to look only to the health care plan for payment"* (Exhibit #8). However, there is no available relief from having to provide the care your doctor is prescribing so long as it is within the capability of the hospital and you have exercised your "right" to self-pay for the care.

Remember, the only enforceable relationship for you is the one you have with your doctor. You haven't signed anything with your managed care insurer and the hospital is literally barred from contracting with you for the cost of the care. Your employer has simply provided a means of paying for the care in your benefit package when and if the insurer agrees to pay. In all other cases, contracted hospitals are required to provide the care free of charge, so long as: 1.) It is an available benefit; 2.) Prescribed by your doctor; 4.) Within the hospital's capability; and, 3.) you have offered to pay for it.

By immediately insisting that your doctor's statements on necessary and appropriate care are a certification of needed care and holding the hospital accountable under the law for providing that care, you strip the insurer of the ability to intervene and reshape your doctor's decision. In other words, you empower the doctor to do his or her job.

Understand that it isn't the doctor's role to mount a fight when your insurer improperly denies coverage. The rights in the law are yours and the doctor isn't an attorney. Moreover, because of the terms and conditions in the Provider Contract that your doctor has been forced to sign, your doctor isn't even in a position to wage this fight effectively. You, on the other hand, have no such constraints. **The right to receive the care prescribed by your doctor is yours. Consequently, it's up to you to enforce it!**

Please don't think that what I am suggesting will lead to smooth sailing. Our family's experience dictates just the opposite. For, while your doctor might not be worried about getting paid for the time devoted to your care, the hospital will be facing tens of thousands of dollars in potentially unpaid expenses if the insurer denies coverage under a fully enforceable Provider Contract. Consequently, like any corporation facing a large loss, they will fight you. They can be counted on to do everything possible to convince you that they are fully within their rights to ignore your doctor whenever your insurance company denies coverage. Unfortunately for them, it just isn't true. Hospitals are bound by both law and their Provider Contracts to provide the care your doctor prescribes, regardless of whether your insurance company agrees to cover the cost. But these rights are yours! And, as the law so often dictates, if you don't press your rights, you lose them. In fact, it's exactly what your insurer is counting on!

Again, I am certainly not saying it will be easy. And I am certainly not trying to tell you what to do. I'm simply trying to share with you what we learned through ten hard years of litigation. How you choose to use the information and exercise your rights has to be your own personal decision. I just wish my family knew as much as I am sharing in this book when we tried to get

Sandy the care she needed! At a minimum, we could have made the critical decisions we faced off knowledge rather than the naïve ignorance the insurance industry and government deliberately foster.

IX.   Why Is This Important? (Why should you and I care)

I would hope the information I have already provided has more than convinced you that what is being done in the name of managed care violates our most basic rights under the Constitution, as well as our sense of fairness and honesty in government. However, with all that being true, there is an element of this issue that can be all too easily overlooked.

While freedom of speech and the press, along with the rights of search and seizure, are often cited as the basis of our freedom, our right of contract, while seldom mentioned, guides our day to day exercise of that freedom. Without the right of contract, we are left naked in our dealings with each other, business, institutions and, most importantly, government. It's the structure that literally allows you to manage your and your family's world and future.

As I have said a number of times, I am not an attorney and I am certainly not trying to slide into that role here. But it's important to understand that without the ability to pay your doctor or hospital for the care you and your family need, there can be "NO" contract between you and your doctor or hospital. And since you can't establish a contract with your doctor or hospital, they owe you "NO" duty other than the avoidance of "provable" negligence. This is huge. It means your doctor and hospital can effectively be an employee of your insurance company, as they most certainly are. And your government is doing everything it can to keep that fact from you. It means that your insurance company is free to deny you the care you and your family need, even if you have the money to pay for it. It means that your insurance company has the power to ration the care you will be allowed to receive with little or no recourse for you. It means that the Republican Party wants to drive us all into private insurance plans where bean counters in hidden offices we will never see have the power to deny us and our loved ones the care we need. All to drive down the national cost of health care, while steadily growing the insurance industry's bottom line. I say again, it's huge!

When I say I had demanded the right to pay for Sandy's care, I would be less than honest if I didn't also mention that I had no intention of surrendering our right to, at some point, pursue Sandy's insurance company for the cost. I was simply separating issues. I was reacting as I would if my automobile insurance company was refusing to cover the cost of repairing a damaged fender. I would tell the body shop to forget about insurance and fix the fender. However, immediately after paying the bill, I would be back to the insurer demanding reimbursement. In other words, I would get the car fixed and then go after the money. I would present the paid bill, we would debate the terms of the policy and then come to some final resolution. All very normal and reasonable in the world of car insurance. In fact, I had long viewed this as normal and reasonable for all forms of insurance.

What took me years of litigation to understand is that HMOs and the other forms of managed care are so different from traditional forms of insurance, that they can't allow this separation of issues to take place. In fact, were it to take place, the outcome is so predictable and dire they can't afford to allow it to even get started.

I failed to understand that managed care had created an entirely new definition for the word "coverage". In traditional insurance, "coverage" defines the conditions under which the insurer is

contractually required reimburse a policyholder for an unanticipated loss or service. However, in managed care, the insurer has no such obligation. The insurer in managed care has designed its Provider Contracts so that the only issue open for determination is whether the provider (doctor or hospital) is allowed to gets paid for the care they are required to supply under law.

In my example of the damaged fender, the debate on whether I qualified for coverage and reimbursement would center on what was owed under the terms of my policy. A policy that would typically make coverage contingent on "how" the damage occurred. If the car was properly parked and then struck by another vehicle, I qualify. However, if I had too much to drink and drove the car into the back wall of my garage, I wouldn't qualify. The same can be said for fire insurance. If your house accidentally catches fire, you have coverage. If you intentionally burn it down, you don't.

Managed care eliminates this whole discussion by stripping the subscriber of their right to directly contract for the care they need. And because insurers: dominate their local market, affiliate to enforce their Provider Contracts nationally and force providers to join their network through sheer market power, there really isn't an alternative source of help when your insurer refuses to approve and pay for the care you need. There certainly isn't a readily available one. In other words, while a subscriber retains the right to contract with a provider outside of the insurer's provider network, that right has little value when insurers won't disclose the extent of their affiliations or the terms and conditions written into their Provider Contracts.

The care we sought for Sandy would not have cost more than about $7,000. And the cost of care for the daughter who committed suicide (see Section III, Our Naïve Pursuit of Justice, page 14) would have been about the same. So, who among us wouldn't take responsibility for $7000 if it meant life or death for ourselves or a loved one?

Yes, most of us with managed care plans get the care we need. Surveys taken by the insurance industry show that most of us are pleased with the care and coverage we receive. But the operative word here is "most" of us. Where care and coverage are denied it's an entirely different picture. People die, or at a minimum, go untreated and never return to full health, all the while being misled and deliberately lied to in support of a system that has no foundation in our laws or sense of justice.

Sandy's death provides the perfect example of what happens when some bean counter in an insurance company's back room is allowed to ration care in order to enhance their own bonus and deliver a better bottom line for the company. While it took years, our naïve pursuit of justice eventually forced Sandy's insurer to produce their internal records on exactly how they made the decision to deny Sandy the care she needed. And, while I hope that by this point the truth won't come as any great surprise, these records showed that the woman who made the decision did so on the basis that *"given Sandy's age and her condition, the cost of the care being prescribed can't be justified."*--- If this isn't an alive and well death-panel that the Conservatives and Republicans are so quick to condemn, then I can't imagine what they are talking about. Of course, these Conservatives and Republicans could be simply doing what Sandy's insurer did throughout all our years of litigation. They simply denied any such decision was ever made. Just like the entire insurance industry steadfastly denies there is anything in their plans that could **"possibly"** prevent a subscriber from paying for necessary health care when an insurance company denies coverage. See Exhibit #7 for an example of just how far these folks are willing

to go to maintain what can only be described as a clear and deliberate lie. In fact, **PLEASE** see Exhibit #7.

Remember, rationing doesn't mean everyone is denied care. It just means that some percentage of lucky souls is singled out for denial. And "death-panel" simply means that once chosen, you will be allowed to die untreated. --- Sandy's case exactly!!!

Simply put, we obviously need affordable health care and the nation needs an affordable health care system. However, your right to freely contract for the care you and your family need, outside the interference of your employer's insurance company, is so fundamental I honestly can't find the words to do it justice. For how serious can we be about "Life, Liberty and the Pursuit of Happiness" if we are willing to blindly surrender our very right to freely access and contract the care we and our families need to pursue Life? All in the name of an affordable national health care system and a more profitable insurance industry!

And lastly, while I have repeatedly condemned the Republican Party and its Conservative Wing for what I believe is a deliberate fraud on the American people, my anger isn't so much focused on what has been done, but rather on my Party's willingness to turn a blind eye to rights of the individual. After all, we are supposedly a Party grounded on Constitutional imperatives that are centered on the rights of the individual and personal freedom. --- How can we then have so lost our way?

X.   How to Make Insurance Work for You (How to beat them every time)

While the way to circumvent what I've been describing is actually quite simple, at least in principle and law, it didn't come quickly or easily to me. It took me the entire ten years of litigation. I was talking with the lead attorney for Aetna at the back of a federal courtroom during a break in what was obviously the end of the line for our case when something he said caused a light bulb to go off in my head.

For ten years I had thought of nothing but how to prove we that had been denied the right to pay for the care prescribed for Sandy. I never climbed out of that box. I was focused solely on proving to the various courts that the actions of Sandy's insurer had forced hospitals to refuse to take our money. I was immersed in the belief that any reasonable person could see that if the hospital was barred from accepting our money, we had been denied our "right" to pay for Sandy's care.

The interesting part was that the attorney was a really nice guy. In fact, he was obviously sympathetic to our position. However, as the attorney for Aetna, he was forced to explain that we needed to withdraw our complaint or face serious financial consequences. Simply put, if we didn't withdraw, at least one of the other parties would be coming at us personally. That's when the light went off in my head. I honestly can't remember exactly why.

However, I can remember almost laughing as I told him that I finally understood what they were doing. I at long last had my answer. The key to accessing care isn't actually paying for it. **It's demanding the "right" to pay for it and the "access" this affords subscribers under law**. I then gave him the following example. I should also note that the gentleman I was speaking with was a black attorney.

When a black American walks into a restaurant in the deep South, he can be certain of getting a meal because the law requires the restaurant to serve him so long as he is willing to pay for the

meal and the restaurant is capable of serving the meal (the menu lists it as an available meal). However, when he finishes his meal, the law says nothing about the restaurant having to bill him or take his money. The restaurant is completely free to provide the meal free of charge. They just have to provide the meal. That is the exact structure of our health care laws. If a properly licensed doctor prescribes care and the patient demonstrates a willingness to pay for that care, the hospital must supply it so long as it is an available service of the hospital. However, if the hospital has been so foolish as to have contracted away its right to bill the patient, that's the hospital's problem, not the patient's. The hospital simply has to provide the care free of charge. It's literally the law in every state in the country.

The look on the attorney's face was one I will never forget. I have to believe that, like me, he had never stepped out of the box to view their well-constructed barriers to accessing care from the back side. --- To come at access and coverage through the backdoor rather than through the front door that they have so carefully prepared. --- To enter through a large chink in their armor.

Let's go back to my restaurant example to be certain all of us understand exactly what I am saying. The black American's right to receive a meal comes from the law's requirement that licensed restaurants must serve whoever enters and requests a meal, so long as the customer is willing to pay for it. --- Period! Now let's say the restaurant hangs a sign on the front door offering free food as part of a one-day promotion. --- Is the restaurant now free to deny people service? No way! --- The law requiring the restaurant to serve all customers equally is unaffected by the restaurant's billing decision. Consequently, so long as a customer enters the restaurant and offers to pay, the restaurant has to serve him. However, when the customer goes to leave, a separate provision of the law bars the restaurant from billing the customer so long as the sign promising free food remains on the door.

Our nation's laws on health care and insurance have the very same structure as our restaurant example. State health care laws and operating licenses require hospitals to provide care to everyone offering to pay so long as it is properly prescribed and the care is within the hospital's capability. However, the combination of state insurance laws, Provider Contracts and the Enrollee Hold Harmless Clause require that the care be provided at no cost to a subscriber, except for coinsurance, copayments and care not listed as an available benefit in a subscriber's benefit package. Simply stated, hospitals must provide the care your doctor is prescribing so long as you demand your right to pay for it. And, if the hospital happens to have signed a Provider Contract with your insurer, the hospital will have no right under the law to bill you. You can simply write "this is a legally unenforceable debt" across any bill the hospital might send you and return it unpaid.

Because insurers feel they have to control the care that subscribers receive, but are barred by law from making these decisions, they contractually require doctors and hospital to "always" provide necessary care. However, these same Provider Contracts have doctors and hospitals voluntarily agreeing to provide this necessary care free of charge anytime the insurer disagrees with what is being prescribed or for a whole list of other reasons written into in these Contracts. It's literally the design of the system. By requiring that doctors and hospitals to provide free care whenever the insurer decides to deny payment, the insurer guarantees that: 1.) The insurer can't be accused of improperly practicing medicine or denying care; and, 2.) Push-come-to-shove, the doctors and hospitals will find a way to support the decisions of the insurer if they want to get paid. It's an absolutely ingenious circumvention of both the spirit and the letter of the law.

Quite obviously, our coming through the backdoor isn't a solution for the nation because the subscriber gets the care free of charge and providers, usually the hospital, gets to eat the cost. However, as I have shown above, this is the intended design of the insurance industry's Provider Contracts and their Enrollee Hold Harmless Clause. Our politicians and the insurers just don't want you to know it. They also believe subscribers are too dumb to ever demand their "right" to pay and the "access" it affords them to free care. In fact, our politicians and the insurance industry are counting on it.

While Provider Contracts make it exceedingly clear that providers are to "agree and comply" with an insurer's determination of "Medically Necessary or Appropriate Care," these Contracts also make it abundantly clear that the providers "must" provide the "Medically Necessary and Appropriate" care that they alone are licensed to determine. Remember, insurers are barred under the law from making any such medical determination. The only decision that they are allowed to make on "Medically Necessary or Appropriate" care is solely for determining the distribution of insurance benefits and controlling costs. Therefore, Provider Contracts don't actually require a hospital to deliver the care an insurer decides is "Medically Necessary or Appropriate." They require the hospital to provide the care your doctor prescribes regardless of whether your insurer is willing to pay for it. Stating this as simply as I can, doctors and hospitals are legally and contractually required to provide all necessary and appropriate care in each and every instance. They just have to provide it free of charge whenever your insurance company chooses to disagree with your doctor, i.e., denies coverage.

Make no mistake, these Provider Contracts have been deliberately written to allow your insurance company to have it both ways. They effectively force providers, including your doctor, to comply with your insurer's non-medical determination of "Medically Necessary and/or Appropriate" care by denying payment, while holding your doctor and hospital accountable for delivering the proper "Medically Necessary and Appropriate care" in all instances.

So, while it's easy to see your doctor and the hospital as innocent victims in this well-constructed scheme, and in many ways they are, you can't afford to if you want to be assured of getting the care you and your family need. Your doctor and hospital have voluntarily signed these Provider Contracts and agreed to keep them secret. Yes, the state and the insurance industry have essentially forced them to sign, but they could have said no. They could have done what their profession demands rather than what is financially expedient. Moreover, there are doctors and hospitals that have done exactly that. Sandy's doctor is an excellent example. Following her inability to appropriately treat Sandy and numerous other patients, she terminated her Provider Contracts and went back to school to become a cosmetic surgeon so that she could treat patients outside any interference from an insurance company. Another example is the Caron Foundation. They are reported to have terminated their Provider Contract with Blue Cross specifically to allow them the freedom to treat patients outside the restrictions of the Enrollee Hold Harmless Clause. In fact, the Foundation's Vice President of Legal told me that terminating their Provider Contract was the only way that they could provide care to patients who had been denied coverage as in Sandy's case. He said the Foundation had exhausted every option in trying to find a way around the Enrollee Hold Harmless Clause to no avail.

The bottom line is that, as subscribers, we have to deal with the system as it exists. And while going through the back door is far from a perfect solution, it's currently the only solution available to subscribers being unfairly denied coverage.

Obviously, the law will vary from state to state. However, there is a common structure. Every state has two separate bodies of laws and regulations that affect a subscriber's ability to access health care. Your state's department of insurance oversees the business of insurance, while the department of health oversees the delivery of health care. This means that your state's department of insurance is responsible for the barriers created by and in support of the Enrollee Hold Harmless Clause. On the other hand, your state's department of health is primarily charged with insuring each of us get the highest possible quality of care. Consequently, our backdoor approach to accessing care focuses on the laws and regulations of your state's department of health, not insurance.

Every hospital must have a state license to operate, and that license must have been approved and issued by your state's department of health. That license stipulates that hospitals can only provide care that has been prescribed by a properly licensed physician. The license further stipulates that the hospital must provide properly prescribed care so long as the hospital has the capability to provide the care and the patient demonstrates a willingness to pay for it.

Please understand that we are not talking about emergency care situations in which hospitals are required to provide care regardless of whether a patient can pay for it. We are talking solely about situations like Sandy's where the doctor is prescribing care or an admission and the hospital is refusing to honor the doctor's decision because the insurer is denying coverage. Consequently, once your doctor has prescribed the care you need, the law and the hospital's license requires the hospital to provide that care <u>so long as you demonstrate a willingness to pay for it</u>. Remember, you have a right to pay. They just can't take your money. But that's their problem. You are fully within your rights to put your offer to pay in writing and threaten to both call the state's attorney general and sue that very day if they don't accept your offer to pay and provide the care prescribed by your doctor and required under law. Confrontational, you bet!

My wife was recently in the hospital for an irregular heartbeat when I happened to walk by the nursing station and overhear a conversation about discharging my wife. This was before we had heard word one from the doctor or had any idea of what was causing my wife's problem. Knowing that a good offense is far better than trying to reverse a decision already made, I leaned over the counter and waited for the nurse to finish the phone call. I then told her that, while I wanted what I was about to say to be taken as openly and friendly as possible, she needed to understand that I knew who she was speaking with and exactly what they were discussing. Furthermore, I said I know more about the subject than anyone in the hospital or probably the state. *"And, if this hospital thinks they are going to discharge my wife before the doctor meets with me and certifies in writing that she is ready for discharge, the hospital is making the biggest mistake of its life because I will be in my attorney's office before the day is out to file suit. So please don't go there, don't take us there!"*

Obviously the poor woman was a bit lost for words, but the doctor was in my wife's room within minutes, full of smiles and assuring me that *"nothing is going to happen until he and I have met and agreed on the proper course of treatment for my wife."* All I ever wanted!

Now that I have convinced you that you need to take control of these situations, or at least I hope I have, let me try to give you a list of some things you can do to get the care you need rather than just a philosophy of confrontation. And please remember, confrontation only works when used as a scalpel, not an ax. It needs to be focused and directed at a specific solution.

Cultivate Your Doctor, for He Is The Door to Accessing Care

Only a properly licensed physician can prescribe health care. So if you can't find a doctor to prescribe the care you need, you will have absolutely no right to receive that care and every hospital and treatment facility will be barred under law from providing it.

Remember, the system is your enemy, not the doctor. You need to win your doctor's willing and active support. And if, for some reason, this can't be done, you need to find another doctor. You need to make the doctor your friend and advocate!!!

When Is Denial of Coverage Most Likely

While most Americans report that they are satisfied with the care and coverage they receive, there are areas of care where this is not likely to be the case and you need to anticipate your insurer denying coverage. These areas are mental health, drug and alcohol rehabilitation, additional days in hospital, all care that can be labeled cosmetic care, all forms of care that your insurer can label experimental, all care that can be somehow linked to an undisclosed precondition and all forms of expensive care for the elderly. In these areas, you need to anticipate a problem and work closely with your doctor to avoid one.

Understand That the Issue Isn't Coverage, It's Whether You "Need" The Care

While only your doctor can prescribe care, the states have passed laws giving insurance companies the authority to determine whether the care your doctor prescribes is "Medically Necessary or Appropriate" for the purpose of insurance and coverage. Therefore, the game your insurer will be playing when they deny coverage is: 1.) Expecting you to believe their doctors can prescribe the care you should receive; 2.) Believing they can force your doctor to change his position over time; and, 3.) Knowing that if they can pull you and your doctor into their review and appeal process, they have won --- the issue always being money not care!

Unfortunately, your doctor will almost never put his or her prescription for care in writing. And even if he or she does, your insurer knows that: 1.) Your doctor has contractually agreed to "comply" with the policies and decisions of the insurer and 2.) Because the hospital has no hope of getting paid, the doctor will eventually be forced to agree with the insurer and the system.

Know The Law Better Than Your Hospital/Doctor

Once your doctor begins to treat you, he or she takes on a duty in law and a professional obligation to prescribe and provide the care you need. However, a hospital doesn't have to admit you unless: 1.) Your doctor has admissions rights; 2.) The care is within the hospital's capability; and, 3.) There is a reasonable expectation the hospital can get paid. The first two requirements are both obvious and essentially met automatically. What neither your insurer nor the hospital will ever tell you, is that if your insurance company refuses to pay for the care your doctor is prescribing, the hospital is bound by its Provider Contract to provide that care free of charge. The fact that the hospital has signed away its right to bill you in no way lessens your right to pay for the care. You just have to demand your right to pay in order to

obligate the hospital, under law, to provide the care being prescribed by your doctor. Consequently, should your insurer refuse to cover this prescribed care, you have every right to **immediately**: 1.) Put your offer to pay in writing; 2.) File an immediate complaint with the state's Attorney General; and, 3.) Threaten to sue the hospital that very day for failing to comply with the laws of the state and the requirements of their license. Knowing, full well that, if ever billed, you are within your rights to refuse the bill as a *"legally unenforceable debt."*

Don't Let The System Get Ahead of You (Anticipate & Listen)

Three years ago, our youngest daughter gave birth to two of the prettiest twin girls we could ever ask for. However, Kris is quite small and the twins were both large healthy babies. As a result, her stomach muscles were badly torn, leaving her with a great deal of discomfort and pain. And while the solution was simple, it's called a tummy-tuck and only available from a cosmetic surgeon, I can't begin to count the number of times the insurer tried to get the term "Cosmetic Surgery" into the record. Cosmetic surgery typically being an elective procedure not available under insurance (not an available benefit/Covered Service). However, what Kris needed was no more elective surgery than surgery to repair the bones in the face of an accident victim. Her insurance company was simply trying to document a means for denying coverage.

Anticipating the problem, I took charge of all correspondence and insured the record never included any reference to cosmetic surgery or an elective procedure. That included what her doctor wrote. Not easy, but doable, because, like in most cases, the doctor was a strong advocate for the care Kris needed! The result was that Kris received the coverage she was due and was able to return to full health. Unfortunately, I have to believe that there is just no way Kris would have gotten coverage if we hadn't anticipated the way her insurer would attempt to deny coverage and cut them off at the pass!

The Threat of Discharge Is Your Constant Enemy

My wife was recently in the hospital for an irregular heartbeat and I happened to overhear the nurse discussing discharging her. Now, neither my wife nor I had met with the doctor or had been given any indication of her condition. So I leaned over the nurse's station and said the following after she finished her phone call. I said *"I want what I am going to say to be taken as openly and friendly as possible. However, I know who you were speaking with and exactly what you were discussing and I know more about the subject than anyone in this hospital or the state. And if this hospital thinks for one moment they are going to discharge my wife before the doctor meets with me and takes direct responsibility for both her care and discharge, the hospital is making the biggest mistake of its life because I will be in my attorney's office to file suit before the day is out. So please don't go there. Don't take us down that road."* I then thanked her for her time and went back to my wife's room. Minutes later the doctor popped into her room all full of smiles and assurances nothing would be done until he and I met and agreed on my wife's condition and what needed to be done.

I have repeated this example to make a point. You will never be part of your insurer's determination of "Medically Necessary or Appropriate" care. That decision will be made by

people you will never be allowed to speak to, let alone meet. Your insurer will review your case daily to determine if you should receive one (1) more day of care. Once that decision is "no", the insurer will inform the hospital and your doctor that further coverage is denied and both the hospital and your doctor will know they won't receive one additional penny for your care and treatment.

The hospital will then explain why you have no choice but to accept termination of care and discharge. And, this is when they get really clever. The hospital will require you to approve your own discharge. Just read the fine print of what they require you to sign. For while they will tell you your doctor has approved the discharge, the doctor is actually only complying with your decision to discharge yourself. The doctor is simply not objecting to your decision.

Of course the hospital will be telling you there is no choice but to be discharged and assuring you that your doctor is in full agreement with the decision. However, watch what happens if you demand to see an order prescribing discharge signed by your doctor. My experience is that everything will go silent while the hospital regroups and looks for support to get you out of the hospital.

Consequently, if you are only looking for an additional day or two in the hospital, as opposed to additional lengthy and expensive treatment, you can almost certainly get this by simply requiring the hospital to produce an "order" for discharge signed by your doctor. The hospital won't get paid, but your doctor isn't likely to sign a recommendation or order for discharge where he or she takes full responsibility for the decision. This would be particularly true for a woman who had given birth and simply wants an additional day or two of hospitalization to recuperate. On the other hand, if it's just for a day or two, you could simply say you don't feel well enough to leave and refuse to go. What are they going to do? Call the police?

Remember, once your insurer denies additional coverage, the game will be played on their court under their rules. Neither the doctor nor the hospital will be paid from that point on and the insurer will know that the lack of payment will, in the end, force the doctor and hospital to agree with the insurer's decision to discharge you or your loved one.

Understand That Transfer to A Nursing Home Equals The Loss of Your Doctor

As a general rule, nursing homes only provide custodial care (essentially room and board). Consequently, there is little chance your doctor will have any rights to attend you or your loved one in a nursing home. Were the doctor to agree to continue to attend you or your loved one without the ability to provide appropriate treatment, the doctor would be opening themselves to significant liability. Not something they are going to want to do!

While I can't prove it, I'm confident insurance companies count on a subscriber's doctor withdrawing from the case when they force the discharge of a patient to a nursing home. The insurer knows the doctor can't follow a patient into a nursing home and they know the home lacks both a license and the ability to treat a patient. Consequently, the insurer can be confident that any appeal of a forced discharge to a nursing home effectively dies with the discharge, as does any request for additional remedial care or treatment. The insurer can simply walk away from the needs and costs of a subscriber and be counted on to do exactly that. Our exact experience with Sandy.

Understand That Providers Close Ranks

Doctors are generally fine people intent on providing you with all the care you need. Hospitals aren't much different. However, both are hostage to an insurance system that creates enormous potential for litigation and awards in millions of dollars. Consequently, these providers can be counted on to avoid this kind of conflict and liability like the plague. That includes insuring that the documented record of a patient's needs supports his or her treatment and discharge. Fortunately for doctors and hospitals, and unfortunately for us, this isn't too difficult because most of what a doctor prescribes is done verbally. So while there will always be some documented decisions, it's highly unlikely there will be any smoking guns. When all the smoke clears, one can be pretty certain the records will show the participants (doctors, hospital and insurer) were in complete agreement on appropriate care and treatment. Furthermore, because the appeal process or any form of litigation is long and complex, any opinions or facts that a subscriber might reasonably count on to contest the written record will almost certainly fade away. --- Pressured providers "will" close ranks!

Act vs. Wait and Hope

As I mentioned earlier, there is a familiar saying among attorneys --- No harm, no foul. It's both a common expression and an underlying principle of law. It's particularly true here. If you fail to <u>immediately</u> press your right to pay for care when unfairly denied coverage, you may very well lose the opportunity to establish any harm or damage. And without harm or damage, there can be no issue. In other words, if you don't act, you can all too easily lose your ability to ever press your right to access necessary health care.

Threating to Sue Is Your Greatest Weapon - <u>Having to Sue Is Failure</u>

While there is much that could be said here, it's not for this book. After ten years in court, I am more than convinced that suing is the last thing you want to do. However, the last thing your insurance company wants is to have the Enrollee Hold Harmless Clause and the many issues it creates brought into question. They certainly won't want our back door approach to coverage debated in open court! However, should you actually sue for the right to pay as we did, you can be assured they will fight you tooth and nail because you will be attacking the entire industry and the very foundation of the managed care business model!

XI.   Definitions You Need to Win

If you are anything like me, you will be tempted to skip this section as simply a list of boring definitions. However, I implore you to not do it here. The fraud I have described in this book is so grounded on the industry's deliberate misuse of critical terms that there is simply no way to understand how subscribers are being denied care without reading this section carefully. Moreover, knowing the "real" definitions of these terms is the only way you will have any chance of understanding what is going on when and if your insurer chooses to deny you the care you or your loved ones need. I ask that you pay particular attention to the following terms: Denial of overage, Medically Necessary or Appropriate Care, Non-Covered Services, Pre-Certification and Utilization Review.

Appeal Process: A process purported to allow subscribers to appeal their insurer's decisions, but intentional lengthy and circuitous to be largely ineffective and a waste of time.

Benefit: Specific care defined as available in the Benefit Package of a Plan, but contingent on the insurer's willingness to pay for it (the determination of willingness to pay being essentially an unrestricted right of the insurer).

Benefit Package: The health care services to be provided to a subscriber by an HMO or similar managed care plan, i.e., the services promised to be available (your Coverage) under your Plan.

Benefit Period: The period of time contractually covered by a subscribers Plan, typically, one calendar year beginning on January 1 of each year and ending on December 31 of the same year.

Coinsurance Amount: A percentage of the allowed charge for a Covered Service (set by a Provider Contract) that is defined in the subscriber's Plan as the subscriber's responsibility. Providers may require the Coinsurance Amount be paid at the time of service.

Copayment Amount: A specific dollar amount defined in the subscriber's Plan as payable by the subscriber for certain Covered Services received during the Benefit Period and a provider is free to require be paid at the time of service. Generally, Copayments Amounts do not apply toward Deductible or Coinsurance Amounts.

Coverage: A term for which the insurance industry uses two (2) very different definitions:

1) Coverage being all the benefits defined as available within the Benefit Package of your Plan, and
2) Denial of Coverage being your insurance company's refusal to approve and pay for care in a particular instance when the care is an available benefit in your Plan's Benefit Package.

Covered Services: The benefits that are available in the Benefit Package of your Plan independent of whether your insurer agrees to approve and pay for them in a particular case.

Deductible Payment: A specific dollar amount defined in the subscriber's Plan as payable by the subscriber for certain Covered Services received during the Benefit Period and the provider is free to require be paid at the time of service.

Denial of Coverage: Contrary to what insurers would like you to believe, this is not a denial of Coverage. It is a refusal to pay for a benefit that is available under the Benefit Package of your Plan. The insurer is simply deciding you either do not need the care or it's too expensive and refusing to pay for it.

Enrollee Hold Harmless Clause: Specific language states required in every Provider Contract that:

1) Bars Providers from billing subscribers for Covered Services,
2) Bars Providers from collecting payments from subscribers for Covered Services, and
3) Bars Providers from contracting privately with subscribers to deliver care the insurer has decided it will not approve or pay for, and
4) Along with the Provider Contract, provides the enforcement mechanism for denying care, i.e., rationing care.

HMO Plan: A Health Care Management Plan offered by an insurance company and usually purchased by an employer or other organization, in which employees or members of the

organization are provided membership in the Plan. As such, the member is only a subscriber or enrollee in the Plan without any ownership in the Plan.

Medically Necessary or Appropriate Care: A term the insurance industry would like you to believe has but one definition. Unfortunately, the insurers, once again, use two very different definitions:

1) The insurer's determination of needed care based on their willingness to pay for a Covered Service in a specific case, and
2) The legal determination of needed care by your (a subscriber's) doctor.

Insurers deliberately confuse the two definitions knowing that doctors and hospitals will be contractually driven to agree with the insurer's decision on appropriate care. --- It is literally the gold mine behind HMO profits and the center of their power to ration care.

Non-Covered Services: Only those services that are specifically excluded from the Benefit Package of your HMO or other managed care Plan, i.e., those services specifically not available under the Plan and your Coverage. Such services are typically limited to elective cosmetic treatments and experimental care.

Pre-Certification: The insurer's process for approving all but emergency care prior to the actual delivery of care. And while the insurance industry would love to have us stop here, the choice of these words speaks volumes in terms of proving the insurance industry is involved in a deliberate fraud aimed at circumventing the law. Remember, only a properly licensed physician can prescribe (certify) the care a patient needs. And once that properly licensed physician (your doctor) certifies what is needed, a hospital must provide that care. It's the law in every state in the country. The only exception is if the care is outside the facility's capability or there is no way for the patient to cover the cost. But, even here, the hospital has some obligation to provide the care by, at a minimum, transferring the patient to another facility willing and able to provide the care the doctor is prescribing. However, if the insurer can intervene prior to the doctor actually "prescribing/certifying" the care a patient needs, they can circumvent the law. In short, the insurer guarantees itself the opportunity to tell the doctor and the hospital in advance that, under the terms of their Provider Contracts, they won't be able to bill anyone for the care the doctor is "considering." And since a doctor isn't likely to force a hospital to provide free care, even if the doctor is willing to go unpaid, the insurer can rest assured the doctor will be changing his or her opinion to conform with that of the insurer. --- Simply put, Pre-Certification isn't a determination of Coverage as your insurer would have you believe. It's the insurer's process for strong-arming your doctor into agreeing with their determination of what is needed and appropriate.

By labeling the process a "Pre-Certification," the insurer asserts that anything your doctor prescribes prior to "Pre-Certification" constitutes no more than preliminary thoughts leading to the doctor's actual "certification/prescription" of necessary and appropriate care. It's a clear violation of the spirit of the law in every state, if not the letter of the law.

Provider Contract: A state mandated contract between the insurance company and all the providers in the insurer's network of approved providers that:

1) Defines the access you will be allowed to have to necessary health care, and
2) You will never be allowed to see. --- **See Exhibit 2 for a representative example and Chapter IV for A Detailed Analysis.**

Rescissions: The insurance industry's process for representing some earlier failure to disclose health care information as a failure to disclose a precondition in order to justify terminating a subscriber's participation in his or her health Plan and avoid the cost of care required to treat a serious illness.

Subscriber: A member or an enrollee in an HMO or other similar form of a managed care Plan, as opposed to a policyholder in a plan. The terms subscriber, enrollee and member have exactly the same meaning and can be used interchangeably.

Uninsured: Individuals without insurance, but with unrestricted access to all necessary and appropriate health care.

Utilization Review: A process in which the insurer has the right, under the terms of its Provider Contracts, to review each patient's case daily and decide whether to provide any additional care. The review can also be retroactive and deny coverage (payment) for care that was properly pre-certified and already rendered to a subscriber. However, in all retroactive denials of coverage, the insurer's Provider Contracts clearly state that the provider (Hospital or Doctor) "*shall not bill or charge Insurer or Subscriber.*" See Section 5. Utilization Review, in Exhibit #2. More specifically, see provisions 5.8, 5.9 and 5.10. Please note that these restrictions on billing subscribers are in addition to the Enrollee Hold Harmless Clause's absolute bar against such billings.

By requiring doctors and hospitals to sign the insurer's Provider Contract, the insurer grants itself the power to deny payment at any time because it is too expensive given its policies and financial objectives. However, to avoid litigation from damaged subscribers, these Provider Contracts make it crystal clear that the provider cannot "*bill or charge*" a subscriber.

I could stop here, but I happened to hear a program by Dr. Sonjay Gupta over the weekend that provides an excellent example of a Utilization Review and how insurers and providers twist the definitions of key terms to serve their own interests.

Dr. Gupta interviewed a woman who had undergone extensive throat surgery to relieve a condition that was seriously restricting her ability to breathe. She explained that her insurance company had pre-certified the procedure and then months later (I believe it was some 9 months after the operation) informed her that they were denying coverage and refusing to pay for the operation. The hospital then billed her for more than a million dollars.

Dr. Gupta's question was "How is this possible?" The woman had done no more than proceed with the care her insurer had agreed to cover. Dr. Gupta said he was completely mystified and promised to devote future programming to the issue.

To answer Dr. Gupta's question, one simply needs to look to the terms and conditions of the Provider Contract that the hospital signed with the woman's insurance company. Of course, as I have said repeatedly, no one is going to willingly make that Provider Contract available. However, rest assured it contains provisions that, for all practical purposes, mirror provisions 5.8, 5.9 and 5.10 in Exhibit #2. In fact, insurers typically publish an entire manual on how these Utilization Reviews are to be conducted. --- The bottom line being that managed care insurance companies (and almost certainly the insurer of Dr. Gupta's guest) use their Provider Contracts to give them almost unlimited power to deny payment to a doctor or hospital whenever the insurer chooses. --- Period!

The only issue open for discussion is whether the hospital had a right to bill Dr. Gupta's guest once coverage was withdrawn, i.e., the insurer had decided to refuse to pay the bill. The answer is an unequivocal "No." However, we are talking about a million dollars. A sum the hospital could be expected to do everything possible to recover. Clearly not something the insurer would relish as it could all too easily involve disclosing the details of their Provider Contracts and the many legal issues they raise.

Fortunately for both the insurer and the hospital there is a simple solution, all be it a deliberate fraud. They need only infer creatively that the insurer's denial of coverage made the operation a "Non-Covered Service". After all, who would think it could be anything else?

By allowing everyone to conclude the woman's operation had become a "Non-Covered Service," the insurer frees the hospital to bill the woman and pursue payment through the courts. Even better for the insurer, they guarantee the matter will be focused on whether they had a right to deny coverage based on their determination of medical necessity and appropriateness. A clear win for the insurer because the woman's managed care Plan provides the insurer this very power. It's a slam dunk.

The answer for Dr. Gupta and his guest was for someone to recognize that the operation the lady received remained a "Covered Service" under law and contract, regardless of what the insurer decided in their Utilization Review. Therefore the hospital had no legal right to bill the woman. The Enrollee Hold Harmless Clause, as well as numerous other provisions in the hospital's Provider Contract, make this point crystal clear. Remember, the Provider Contract and the Enrollee Hold Harmless Clause are mandated by state law, so there is no way the hospital can deny they exist. Dr. Gupta's guest should have marked the hospital's bill a "legally unenforceable debt" and sent it back unpaid. At a bare minimum, she, or her attorney, should have demanded the hospital produce a copy of their Provider Contract to prove they had a legal right to bill her. Imagine the mess that would have created for the hospital as their Contract almost certainly bars any and all such billing while prohibiting the hospital from disclosing the details of the Contract.

And so we come once again to the purpose of this book. There is just no way Dr. Gupta's guest could reasonably be expected to stand against the attorneys pursuing her for a million dollars. These are very smart people and they have executed this type of deception so many times that they are not only experts at it, but brash and intimidating as well. Furthermore, I have yet to find a private attorney with enough understanding of the system to provide the help the woman needed. Remember, I was immersed in this mess for ten years and never found an attorney with sufficient understanding to help. Hopefully our experience and this book will not only answer Dr. Gupta's question, but throw some much needed light on the entire issue!

XII.   Summing Up the Issue & Solution

As I have done throughout the book, I'm going to use the term HMO to represent the many forms of managed care available in the market. We can do this because HMOs are by far the most common form of managed care and the others take a very similar approach to the individual subscriber and the delivery of health care. Furthermore, I will be using the term "provider" to include not only doctors and hospitals, but all suppliers of skilled health care.

In order to protect their authority to regulate insurance, the states have adopted recommendations of the National Association of Insurance Commissioners (NAIC) that require HMOs to have a Provider Contract with every provider in their broad network of approved providers and that these Contracts must contain a provision known as the Enrollee Hold Harmless Clause. And while these requirements appear to have provided the protection the states were seeking, the requirements have given HMOs the power to effectively deny care at will in pursuit of lower costs and a stronger bottom line.

Stating the problem as simply as possible, by requiring providers to sign Provider Contracts with HMOs, the states have empowered the HMOs to dictate exactly when and if a provider will get paid for the care they supply to a subscriber while holding the provider absolutely responsible for delivering the correct "Necessary and Appropriate" care at all times. In other words, the only way for a provider to get paid is to "support" the HMO's decisions on care and coverage. Consequently, HMOs don't actually deny care, they simply make it impossible for a provider to get paid if they render care the HMO refuses to approve.

But what if the subscriber simply elects to step outside the coverage of his or her HMO insurance and contract directly for the cost of the care the HMO is refusing to cover. Unfortunately, the recommendations of the NAIC completely eliminate this option. In order to preserve the authority of the states to regulate insurance, the language in NAIC's Enrollee old Harmless Clause (a must for all Provider Contracts) has providers surrendering any and all right to privately contract outside the terms and conditions of their Provider Contract.

The bottom line is that the states have placed provisions in their laws that: 1.) Bar providers from getting paid unless they support the decisions of an HMO and 2.) Eliminate any and all right of providers to contract outside the terms and conditions of an HMO's Provider Contract and Enrollee Hold Harmless Clause. And if this were not enough of an affront to our sense of law and justice, every involved party has not only kept this a deep dark secret, but actively worked to confuse and mislead subscribers on the issue. They have deliberately confused and misled subscribers to the point of watching them die without the care they are due under the health care laws of the states and the terms and conditions of the applicable Provider Contracts! --- The rationing of necessary health care at its very best!

The icing on the cake is that these Provider Contracts and HMO plans have subscribers surrendering their right to necessary care without "any" process or informed consent. In fact, subscribers don't even have any ownership in their HMO plans as the plans are written by the HMOs and almost always purchased by the subscriber's employer. The subscriber is simply being granted participation in his or her employer's contracted plan.

Fortunately, there is a gaping hole in the system that the states have created and the HMOs have taken to the bank. It's a wide open backdoor if you know where and how to look. The very same state laws and Provider Contracts also make it absolutely clear that: 1.) Subscribers have every right to pay for properly prescribed "necessary and appropriate health care; 2.) Providers are absolutely required to provide it: and, 3.) Providers must provide it free of charge if the HMO refuses to provide coverage. All a subscriber has to do to obligate a hospital to provide the care his or her HMO is refusing to approve is to offer to pay knowing that, so long as the hospital is within the insurer's network of approved providers, the hospital is legally barred from ever sending the subscriber a bill or collecting the subscriber's money. You just have to demand your

right to pay, knowing they can't bill you, and hold the hospital accountable under law and the terms of their Provider Contract for delivering the care your doctor is prescribing.

This is what congressional politicians, state governments, the insurance industry, and hospitals want desperately to keep you from understanding! This is what took the Lobb family ten years of litigation and the death of Sandra Lobb to discover. It's what the Republicans (particularly Conservatives), state governments, the insurance industry, your HMO insurer and hospitals affiliated with HMOs desperately want to keep from you!

It's exactly what: 1.) The Federal Government (both sides of the aisle) doesn't want you to know in order to drive down the national cost of health care; 2.) The Republican Party doesn't want you to know in order to privatize Medicare; 3.) Your state government doesn't want you to know in order to avoid federal intervention in the regulation of insurance; 4.) The insurance industry doesn't want you to know because it threatens their entire industry; 5.) Your insurer doesn't want you to know because it threatens their bottom line; and, 6.) Doctors and hospitals are specifically barred from telling you because it interferes with your constitutional right to freely access health care! --- Taken collectively, these efforts to hide what can only be described as the illegal rationing of necessary care and the existence of all too real death panels constitute "The Great Health Care Fraud" described in the book. A fraud that I have repeatedly described as masterfully constructed!!!

If you have HMO insurance, you always have coverage for necessary health care. The only question is who (HMO, hospital or doctor) is legally required to pay for it? --- **Clearly not you**!

And lastly, I need to remind the reader and anyone who comes in contact with the contents of this book, that I am not an attorney, nor am I representing myself as an expert on the laws that affect the delivery of health care and insurance in the United States. The book is solely the author's attempt to share what ten years of litigation and the death of Sandra Lobb appears to have taught him. Consequently, everything described in the book should be reviewed by a competent attorney prior to any individual putting it into practice, or relying on it as accurate, for the delivery of necessary health care or insurance.

Exhibits

1. The Enrollee Hold Harmless Clause
2. Representative Provider Contract
3. Pennsylvania Regulation On HMO Insolvency
4. ERISA Preemption Manual for State Health Policy Makers
5. Maryland Attorney General Statement
6. Affidavit Defining Covered Services
7. Aetna's Acknowledgment You Can't Pay
8. Blue Cross Letter to Art Hershey

#1: <u>Enrollee Hold Harmless</u> Clause (It's in every Provider Contract)

Hospital/Doctor agrees that in no event, including but not limited to non-payment by Insurance Company, Insurance Company's insolvency or breach of this agreement, shall Hospital, one of its subcontractors, or any of its employees or independent contractors bill, charge, collect a deposit from, seek compensation, remuneration or reimbursement from, or have any recourse against a Subscriber or persons other than the insurance company acting on behalf of Subscriber for Covered Services provided pursuant to this Agreement. This provision shall not prohibit the collection of coinsurance, co-payments or charges for Non-Covered Services. Hospital/Doctor further agrees that (1) this provision shall survive the termination of this Agreement regardless of the cause giving rise to termination and shall be construed to be for the benefit of the Subscribers, and that (2) this provision supersedes any oral or written contrary agreement now existing or hereafter entered into between Hospital/Doctor and Subscribers or persons acting on their behalf. Hospital/Doctor may not change, amend or waive this provision without prior written consent of the Insurance Company. Any attempt to change, amend or waive this provision are void.

#2: **Representative Provider Contract**

The following is a representative Provider Contract without its mundane boilerplate provisions. It is not a copy of any specific insurer's provider contract to avoid the charge of disclosing secret proprietary information. However, it is an accurate representation the provider contracts insurance companies use to restrict the freedom of doctors and hospitals to deliver appropriate care to subscribers while empowering the insurance company's ability to deny coverage.

THIS PARTICIPATING PROVIDER AGREEMENT ("Agreement"), is made and entered into between **INSURER** and **HOSPITAL/DOCTOR** to establish terms and conditions for the rendering and payment of services to Subscribers in accordance with insurance plans issued by **INSURER**.

NOW, THEREFORE, in consideration of the premises and mutual covenants contained herein and other good and valuable consideration, the receipt and sufficiency of which are hereby acknowledged, it is mutually agreed by and between the Parties as follows:

ARTICLE 1

DEFINITIONS

For the purpose of this Agreement, the following definitions shall apply:

1.1   CHARGES – The Hospital's/Doctor's itemized listing of the rates it charges for patient services.

1.2   COVERED SERVICES – The services listed in a Subscriber's insurance benefit package AND rendered to the Subscriber.

1.3   NON-COVERED SERVICES – The services that are defined as NOT available services in the Subscriber's insurance Plan and benefit package (*typically limited to elective cosmetic surgery and experimental treatments*).

1.4   NETWORK – The participating providers with which Insurer, its affiliates, contractors and subcontractors has contracted to furnish COVERED SERVICES under a subscriber benefit package issued by Insurer.

1.5   ENROLLEE – A subscriber who is eligible to receive COVERED SERVICES under an insurance Plan and benefit package issued by Insurer.

1.6   SUBSCRIBER – An enrolled and eligible individual, or dependents, who has satisfied the criteria for benefits under an insurance Plan provided and administered by Insurer.

1.7   EMERGENCY – A sudden onset of acute medical or psychiatric symptoms of sufficient severity, that in the absence of immediate medical attention, could result in: 1.) Permanent injury to the subscriber, or 2.) Cause other serious medical or psychological consequences.

1.8   EMERGENCY CARE – Medically necessary care and services and supplies provided to a subscriber in an emergency.

1.9   MEDICALLY NECESSARY or APPROPRIATE CARE – The requirement that Covered Services are required, in the opinion of: (1.) the primary care physician, or the referred

specialist, as applicable, consistent with Insurer's policies, coverage requirements and utilization guidelines; and (2.) Insurer, in order to diagnose and treat a subscriber, as applicable, and:

    a. Are provided in accordance with established standards and practices;
    b. Are required to improve the subscriber's health and health outcome; and
    c. Are as cost-effective as any available and approved alternative.

SECTION 2. PROVISION of COVERED SERVICES

2.1   Hospital/Doctor shall furnish Medically Necessary or Appropriate Services to eligible Subscribers in accordance with the terms and conditions of the Subscriber's insurance Plan and this Agreement.

2.2   Hospital/Doctor shall be solely responsible for the quality of Covered Services rendered to Subscriber. Hospital/Doctor further acknowledges that any action taken by Insurer pursuant to utilization management or cost containment in no way absolves Hospital/Doctor of the responsibility to provide appropriate care to Subscriber.

2.3   Covered Services shall be rendered a Subscriber by Hospital/Doctor without any advance deposit or other charge to Subscriber, except for copayments and deductible payments described in the Subscriber's insurance Plan.

2.4   Doctor/Hospital agrees to render Covered Services in accordance with: (a) all terms and conditions set forth in this Agreement, (b) all applicable laws and regulations, and (c) the same manner and timeliness as all other patients without regard to reimbursement.

SECTION 3. PAYMENT for SERVICES RENDERED

3.1   Hospital/Doctor shall submit claims for Covered Services no more than 90 days from the date the Covered Services are rendered.

3.2   Insurer shall pay Hospital/Doctor in accordance with the rates set herein for Medically Necessary and Appropriate Covered Services rendered Subscribers per the terms and conditions set forth in this Agreement.

3.3   Covered Services approved by Insurer and rendered by Hospital/Doctor shall be paid as provided herein, UNLESS: (a) excluded as a Non-Covered Service by a Subscribers insurance Plan and benefit package, (b) Insurer informs Hospital/Doctor that a given service is not a Covered Service, or (c) Insurer determines the service to be not Medically Necessary or Appropriate.

3.4   If all or any part of the Covered Services rendered a Subscriber by Hospital/Doctor was not ordered by a properly licensed health professional operating within the scope of that license, the Hospital/Doctor shall not bill or charge either Insurer or the Subscriber for that portion of the Covered Service.

3.5   Hospital/Doctor shall accept payments made by Insurer for Covered Services, including non-payment, as payment in full for all Covered Services rendered to a Subscriber and shall comply with the Employee Hold Harmless provision set forth below. The Insurer's payment, including non-payment, shall therefore discharge all obligation of Subscriber for Covered Services.

3.6   In the event Insurer makes an incorrect payment or an overpayment to Hospital/Doctor, Hospital/Doctor agrees to refund or reimburse such amounts within five (5) business days. If

Hospital/Doctor fails to refund or reimburse an overpayment, Hospital/Doctor hereby authorizes Insurer to withhold or offset future payments against amounts owed Hospital/Doctor.

SECTION 4. BILLING

4.1   Hospital/Doctor agree to submit bills to Insurer for Covered Services by the later of: (a) ninety days following the date Insurer issues billing approval to Hospital/Doctor or (2) ninety days following the last day of the calendar year in which the Subscriber was discharged from the hospital or ended treatment. If Hospital/Doctor fails to submit billing within this defined period, Insurer shall not be responsible for payment for those Covered Services and Hospital/Doctor shall not bill Subscriber for those Covered Services.

4.2   Insurer agrees to exercise its best efforts to pay appropriate claims for Covered Services within thirty (30) days of receipt of such claims.

SECTION 5. UTILIZATION REVIEW

5.1   All Covered Services rendered to Subscriber by Hospital/Doctor are subject to a medical and utilization review by Insurer or its designee.

5.2   Hospital/Doctor shall notify Insurer of all elective inpatient care to be rendered to a subscriber prior to admission or rendering such elective care.

5.3   Hospital/Doctor shall notify Insurer of all emergency admissions of Subscribers within one (1) business day of such admission.

5.4   Hospital/Doctor shall pre-certify all non-emergency admissions of Subscribers prior to admission by obtaining Insurer's approval of the Medical Necessity or Appropriateness of the admission and proposed length of stay.

5.5   Hospital/Doctor agrees Insurer shall not approve an inpatient admission until all necessary information is provided Insurer.

5.6   Where pre-certification is required but not performed, any and all services and days of care rendered prior to Insurer's pre-certification and approval shall not be billed or charged to Insurer or Subscriber.

5.7   Hospital/Doctor agrees Insurer shall review the Medical Necessity or Appropriateness of an inpatient admission or course of treatment on a daily basis and free to find such admission or course of treatment not Medically Necessary or Appropriate.

5.8   Whenever the Insurer's review of Medically Necessary or Appropriate determines a particular inpatient admission or course of treatment is not Medically Necessary or Appropriate, Hospital/Doctor shall not bill or charge Insurer or Subscriber for that denied stay or treatment. Hospital/Doctor further agrees such reviews and denials can be retroactive and reverse earlier approvals by Insurer or Insurer's designee.

5.9   Whenever an admission or some portion of an admission is determined by Insurer to be not Medically Necessary or Appropriate or other requirements set forth herein are not met, the entire admission shall be denied and the Hospital/Doctor shall not bill or charge Insurer or Subscriber for any services associated with such denied stay or treatment.

5.10   Should Insurer determine a requested admission or course of treatment is not Medically Necessary or Appropriate and Hospital/Doctor nonetheless provides that admission or course of treatment, Hospital/Doctor shall not bill or charge Insurer or Subscriber for any related costs associated with that denied admission or treatment.

SECTION 6. EMPLOYEE HOLD HARMLESS

6.1   Hospital/Doctor agrees that in no event, including but not limited to non-payment by Insurer, Insurer's insolvency or breach of this Agreement, shall Hospital/Doctor, one of its subcontractors, or any of its employees or independent contractors bill, charge, collect a deposit from, seek compensation, remuneration or reimbursement from, or have any recourse against a Subscriber, or persons other than Insurer acting on behalf for services provided pursuant to this Agreement. This provision shall not prohibit the collection of coinsurance, copayments or charges for non-Covered Services. Hospital/Doctor further agrees that (1) this provision shall survive the termination of this Agreement regardless of the cause giving rise to the termination and shall be construed to be for the benefit of the Subscriber, and that (2) this provision supersedes any oral or written contrary agreement now existing or hereinafter entered into between Hospital/Doctor and Subscriber or persons acting on their behalf.

SECTION 7. CONFIDENTIALITY AND DISCLOSURE

7.1   Hospital/Doctor agree not to disclose any information pertaining to business conducted by Insurer, including, but not limited to the payments for Covered Services. Hospital/Doctor further agrees that all such information shall be considered confidential and proprietary and unless required by law, shall not be disclosed, except as otherwise approved by written consent of Insurer.

7.2   Hospital/Doctor specifically acknowledge and agree that a breach of the foregoing provisions will cause Insurer irreparable harm and that the remedy at law for any such breach will be inadequate and that Insurer, in addition to any other relief available to it, shall be entitled to equitable relief and temporary and permanent injunctive relief without the necessity of proving actual damages or posting any bond whatsoever.

SECTION 8. INDEMNIFICATION

8.1.1   Hospital/Doctor agrees to indemnify and hold harmless Insurer from any suit, cost, claim or expense, including, but not limited to, the cost of defense incurred by Insurer as a result of negligent actions or breach of this Agreement by Hospital/Doctor or their employees, contractors or subcontractors in connection with rendering Covered Services pursuant to this Agreement.

SECTION 9. TERM

9.1   This Agreement shall commence as of the date hereof and shall continue for three (3) years, and thereafter shall automatically renew for successive terms of one (1) year. Notwithstanding the foregoing, this Agreement shall not be effective until approved by State Department of Insurance/Health.

SECTION 10. TERMINATION

10.1   Either party may terminate this Agreement by providing the other party with not less than 60 days prior written notice.

10.2   Insurer may immediately terminate this Agreement if, in its sole opinion, Hospital/Doctor fails to comply with any Insurer Policies or Procedures and such failure would reasonably have a material adverse effect on Insurer.

10.3   Insurer may immediately terminate this Agreement if, in its sole opinion, Hospital/Doctor are in breach of any portion of this Agreement and failed to cure such Breach within 30 days of written notification by insurer.

10.4   In the event Hospital/Doctor is providing services to a Subscriber as of the date of termination of this Agreement, Hospital/Doctor shall continue to furnish those services and facilities contemplated to that Subscriber and all other Subscribers who were receiving such services on the date of termination. Hospital's/Doctor's right to receive reimbursement for such Covered Services shall continue to be governed by the applicable terms of this Agreement. This provision shall survive the termination of this Agreement for any reason.

SECTION 11. APPEAL OF UTILIZATION REVIEW DETERMINATIONS

11.1   Hospital/Doctor has the right to appeal an adverse determination by Insurer or its designee on the Medical Necessity or Appropriateness of any requested inpatient admission, length of stay or course of treatment.

11.2   Hospital/Doctor agree to comply with Insurer's policies, procedures and all final determinations of appropriate care and coverage

11.3   Hospital/Doctor agrees decisions by the Insurer's Appeals Panel shall be final, binding and non-appealable for all parties.

IN WITNESS WHEREOF, the undersigned have executed this Agreement on the date set forth below.

INSURANCE COMPANY   HOSPITAL/DOCTOR

By: _____   By: _____

Date _____   Date _____

#3: <u>Pennsylvania Regulation on HMO Insolvency</u>

The following excerpt from the Pennsylvania Code provides clear proof that the State of Pennsylvania is intentionally misleading subscribers when its Department of Insurance describes the Enrollee Hold Harmless Clause as merely a limited ban on billing intended to prevent balance billing by providers. As shown in the excerpt, their own regulations clearly state the Clause is an absolute ban on billing for the purpose of insolvency protection.

Subchapter G. PROTECTION AGAINST INSOLVENCY

Sec.

Source

The provisions of this Subchapter G adopted March 13, 1992, effective March 14, 1992, 22 Pa.B. 1178, unless otherwise noted.

§ 301.121. Protections against insolvency.

(a) A new certificate of authority filing shall include procedures to be implemented to meet the requirements for protection against insolvency.

(b) Requirements for protection against insolvency include:

(1) For new plans filing for a certificate of authority, a minimum initial net worth of $1.5 million.

(2) For every operational HMO, minimum net worth equal to the greater of $1 million or 3 months uncovered health care expenditures for Pennsylvania enrollees as reported on the most recent financial statement filed with the Commissioner. A dedicated funding commitment, such as an irrevocable letter of credit or other instrument from a parent company, may be considered in assessing net worth, if approved by the Commissioner. This commitment would not be considered a substitute for a capital infusion needed to obtain a positive net worth.

(c) Existing HMOs have 4 years to meet the net worth requirements, in increments of $250,000 as of January 1 of each year. The plan is required to include the uncovered expenses amount, if applicable, in the fifth year.

(d) Interest expenses relating to the repayment of a fully subordinated debt are

considered a covered expense.

(e) Fully subordinated debt is not considered a liability.

(f) An HMO shall deposit with the Commissioner cash, securities or a bond, or an acceptable combination, which has a value of at least $100,000. The deposit shall cover administrative costs in the event of liquidation.

(g) The deposit, as required in subsection (f), is an admitted asset of the HMO in the determination of net worth.

(h) Income from deposits is an asset of the organization. An HMO that has made a securities deposit could withdraw that deposit or a part thereof after making a substitute deposit of cash, securities, or a combination of these, or other instruments of equal amount and value.

(i) The Commissioner may reduce or eliminate the deposit requirement if the HMO deposits with the State Treasurer, the Commissioner or other official body of the state of the HMO's domicile for the protection of all subscribers and enrollees of the HMO, wherever located, cash, acceptable securities or surety, and delivers to the Commissioner a certificate to that effect, authenticated by the appropriate state official holding the deposit.

(j) An HMO investment is subject to the investment provisions for a stock life company in sections 404.1 and 404.2 of The Insurance Company Law of 1921 (40 P. S. § § 504.1 and 504.2).

§ 301.122. Hold harmless.

A contract between an HMO and a participating provider of health care services shall include a provision to the following effect:

"(Provider) hereby agrees that in no event, including, but not limited to non-payment by the HMO, HMO insolvency or breach of this agreement, shall (Provider) bill, charge, collect a deposit from, seek compensation, remuneration or reimbursement from, or have any recourse against subscriber/enrollee or persons other than HMO acting on their behalf for services listed in this Agreement. This provision shall not prohibit collection of supplemental charges or copayments on the HMO's or provider's behalf made in accordance with the terms of the applicable agreement between the HMO and subscriber/enrollee.
"(Provider) further agrees that (1) the hold harmless provisions herein shall survive the termination of the (applicable Provider contract) regardless of the cause giving rise to termination and shall be construed to be for the benefit of the HMO subscriber/enrollee and that (2) this hold harmless provision supersedes any oral or written contrary agreement now existing or hereafter entered into between (Provider) and subscriber/enrollee or persons acting on their behalf.
"Any modification, addition, or deletion to the provisions of this section shall become effective on a date no earlier than fifteen (15) days after the Secretary of Health has received written notice of such proposed changes."

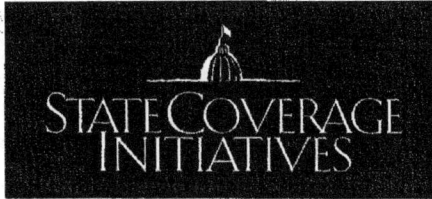

ERISA PREEMPTION MANUAL FOR STATE HEALTH POLICY MAKERS

by Patricia Butler

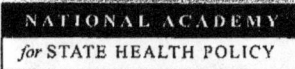
ALPHA CENTER

NATIONAL ACADEMY
for STATE HEALTH POLICY

Provider contract
standards should be
held not to relate to
ERISA plans because
they do not mandate
an employee plan's
structure to the same
extent as any-willing-
provider laws.

inconsistent conclusions about whether ERISA preempts these laws. Although the current weight of authority favors preemption, the Fifth Circuit's secondary holding in the *Texas Pharmacy* case suggests that state laws directed only at insurers might survive an ERISA challenge.[53] Even if a court is not persuaded by the more creative arguments of *American Drug Stores*[54] that AWP laws do not relate to ERISA plans because an ERISA plan could self-insure to avoid the state law, a state AWP law could be saved from preemption by: 1) applying only to entities conducting the business of insurance (which should include HMOs, despite contrary court opinions); 2) making its terms a mandatory part of insurance policies (rather than a mandate on insurance companies); 3) not indicating a purpose to benefit providers by allowing them to participate in health plan networks; and 4) not referring to ERISA plans (even to exempt them from the law's reach). The *UNUM* decision is of little help in defending AWP laws in states where the courts hold that HMOs are not insurers because these laws cannot meet the initial "common sense" test of insurance regulation.

2. Provider contract terms

Concerned over allegations that managed care plans prohibit physicians from freely discussing with patients treatment options that the plan may not cover, many state legislatures have prohibited so-called "gag clauses" in plan-provider contracts despite some question as to whether they exist.[55] Some states also prohibit plans from requiring providers to indemnify them for plan errors. These types of laws have rarely been challenged, but a Texas district court held that ERISA preempts them because they directly affect ERISA plan administrators' discretion in structuring the plan and are not saved as insurance regulation because they apply to HMOs that are not insurers.[56] This reasoning raises the prospect that ERISA might be held to preempt not only these more recent plan-provider contract terms but also the requirement in most state HMO licensing laws that HMOs must prohibit providers from seeking remuneration from enrollees if the plan fails to pay. This "hold harmless" provision is designed to protect plan enrollees from being asked to pay for services if the plan becomes insolvent and is typically used in lieu of insurance "guaranty funds" that pay claims of insolvent indemnity insurers. States may want to require that these provider-enrollee, hold harmless guarantees be part of plan-enrollee contracts in order to better defend them as insurance regulation.

The Texas court's decision invalidating these provider contract terms appears inconsistent with current preemption principles. Provider contract review has been a core activity of HMO regulation in many states because of its impact on the delivery of services to enrollees. Provider contract standards should be held not to relate to ERISA plans because they do not mandate an employee plan's structure to the same extent as AWP laws. Under an AWP law, an ERISA plan arguably cannot achieve cost and quality goals available in an insurer's limited network plan. Provider-patient communications or provider-plan indemnity arrangements would have an insignificant impact on an ERISA plan administrator's ability to contract for cost-effective health coverage. Even if a court were to hold that they relate to ERISA plans, standards prohibiting gag clauses or holding *patients* harmless from providers' unpaid bills should be saved on the ground that they primarily benefit policyholders. Standards chiefly benefitting providers, like the plan indemnity provisions, might be harder to justify as insurance regulation.

3. Provider risk-sharing limits

Managed care companies often attempt to control service use and therefore plan costs by sharing risk with contracting providers. They may pay providers a fixed fee for agreeing to deliver cover-

#5: <u>Maryland Attorney General Statement</u>

The following is extracted from a longer letter from the Maryland Attorney on the ability of providers to bill subscribers subject to state statutes on HMOs and the Enrollee Hold Harmless Clause.

January 28, 2005

To: The Honorable Sharon Grosfeld
Maryland Senate

The State HMO law sets forth the statutory basis for the concept of the HMO, under which a member pays a periodic fee to the HMO in return for the HMO's promise to provide or finance health care services for the member without further charge, except for co-payments or deductibles set forth in the HMO plan. See *Riemer v. Columbia Medical Plan*, Inc., 358 Md. 222, 228-31, 747A.2d 677 (2000); Annotated Code of Maryland, Health-General Article ("HG"), §19-701 *et seq*. A key component of this arrangement is the "hold harmless" clause that appears in any agreement between an HMO and a provider. In particular, the HMO law requires that:

> The hold harmless clause shall provide that the provider may not, *under any circumstances*, including nonpayment of moneys due the providers by the [HMO], insolvency of the [HMO], or breach of the provider contract, bill, charge, collect a deposit, seek compensation, remuneration or reimbursement from, or have any recourse against the [HMO] member … for services provided in accordance with the provider contract.

HG §19-710(i)(2) (emphasis added). Copayments, coinsurance, and charges for services not included in the HMO plan may be excluded from this contractual prohibition. HG §19-710(i)(3).

The statute buttresses this contractual provision by prohibiting health care providers from charging members of an HMO for a "covered service provided to the member. In particular, the State HMO law provides:

(1)Except [for certain copayments and coinsurance], individual enrollees and subscribers of [HMOs] … shall not be liable to any health care provider for any covered services provided to the enrollee or subscriber.

> (2)(i) A health care provider … may not collect or attempt to collect from any subscriber or enrollee any money owed to the health care provider by [an HMO] …

> (ii) A health care provider … may not maintain any action against any subscriber or enrollee to collect or attempt to collect any money owed to the health care provider by [an HMO] …

HG §19-701(p). Essentially, a "covered service" is a "health care service included in the benefit package of the [HMO] …" HG §19-710(d). Thus, "subscribers or members owe no debt to any health care provider (*i.e.*, any doctor, hospital, etc.) for any covered services." *Riemer*, 358 Md. at 244. An HMO member remains liable for copayments and coinsurance as provided in the HMO plan.

J Joseph Curran, Jr.
Attorney General

#6: Affidavit Defining Covered Services

AFFIDAVIT OF HOWARD W. McINTYRE, JR.

COMMONWEALTH OF PENNSYLVANIA)
) SS.
COUNTY OF CHESTER   )

Before me, the undersigned a Notary Public of the Commonwealth of Pennsylvania, appeared HOWARD W. McINTYRE, JR., being duly sworn according to law, did depose and say as follows:

1.   I am presently retired and reside at 341 Lees Bridge Road, Nottingham, Pa 19362.

2.   Prior to my retirement, I was a licensed independent agent in the insurance industry for approximately 19 years. Prior to that, I was employed by Metropolitan Life Insurance Company for 22 years. In total, I worked 41 years (1958 – 1999) for the insurance industry.

3.   During those 41 years, I received numerous awards and commendations for my knowledge and performance. I am a graduate of the Life Underwriting Course Parts 1 and 2 and was licensed to sell health care insurance, including group plans, in the state of Pennsylvania.

4.   My career afforded me extensive experience in all forms of insurance, including health care insurance. More specifically, this experience included writing policies, paying claims, and investigating the many types of issues that arise form the broad range of policies and plans available from the insurance industry. Consequently, I was required to

have a full understanding of the terms, conditions and policies used by the insurance industry to write and administer policies/plans.

5.   While there are clearly many differences between healthcare insurance, life insurance and the many other forms of insurance, one thing they all have in common is their approach to the definition of a "Covered Service or Covered Benefit" (hereinafter "Covered Service/Benefit"). Contrary to what one might intuitively believe, the term "Covered Service/Benefit" is reserved for contractually defining the benefit package available under a particular policy or plan and NOT what an insurer has actually agreed to pay for in a particular instance. In other words, a "Covered Service/Benefit" is what the policy/plan defines as contractually available contingent upon the terms and conditions in a policy/plan.

6.   For example, if a man has a fire insurance policy on his home, the policy will provide reimbursement for fire damage as a "Covered Service/Benefit". However, if an investigation determines the man intentionally lit a fire, coverage will be denied per the terms and conditions in the policy.

7.   Or if a man takes out a life insurance policy, the policy will provide a payment upon death as a "Covered Service/Benefit". However, if an investigation determines he failed to disclose a pre-existing terminal illness, coverage will be denied per the terms and conditions in the policy.

8.   Or if a man purchases health care insurance, the policy will provide a set of specific health care services as "Covered Services/Benefits" of the policy/plan. However, if the insurer determines a requested "Covered Service/Benefit" is not "Medically Necessary", coverage will be denied per the terms and conditions in the policy/plan.

9.   In all three examples, the definition of a "Covered Service/Benefit" remains unchanged by the insurer's refusal to pay, i.e., denial of coverage.

10.   "Non-Covered Services", "Uncovered Services" and "Uncovered Benefits" (hereinafter "Uncovered Services") are equivalent contractual terms reserved by the insurance industry for defining services and benefits that are NOT in the benefit package of a policy/plan. Consequently, they are services/benefits that are outside any consideration for payment/coverage and literally outside the contractual relationship between an insurer and a policyholder.

11.   These various contractual terms used by the insurance industry for defining a benefit package are best viewed as simply "Covered Services" as opposed to "Uncovered Services". "Covered Services" being the services/benefits specifically listed as included in a benefit package and "Uncovered Services" being the services/benefits specifically listed as NOT included in a benefit package. Again, the definitions of these two terms are NOT influenced by an insurer's decision on whether to pay a particular claim. In fact, because they are contractual definitions, they cannot be changed without revising the actual language in the applicable policy/plan.

12.   Consequently, when an insurer denies coverage for a "Covered Service, the insurer is simply denying a claim per the applicable terms and conditions in the policy/plan. When an insurer denies coverage for an "Uncovered Service", the insurer is claiming the service or benefit is literally outside the contractual agreement established by the applicable policy/plan.

13.   The entire insurance industry has been built upon this simple but rigorous contractual foundation.

79

14. Any attempt to convey the thought that a "Covered Service" becomes an "Uncovered Service" when an insurer denies payment or coverage for a particular "Covered Service/Benefit", can only be seen as a deliberate attempt to mislead or the product of complete ignorance on the practices of the insurance industry.

_____
HOWARD W. McINTYRE, JR

SWORN TO AND SUBSCRIBED before me, a Notary Public, of the State and County aforesaid, this _13_ day of _Sept_____, 2006

_____
NOTARY PUBLIC

#7: Aetna's Acknowledgment You Can't Pay

The following is an e-mail conversation between Rich Mangini, an employee of Cameron's Hardware & Supply, Inc. and J. P. Kearney, a corporate account manager for Aetna Health Care Insurance.

++

April 26, 2006

We are a medium sized business that provides your health care insurance as part of our benefit package. Recently, one of our employees asked whether Pennsylvania law requires an employee to look only to his or her health care policy/plan for payment of care included in the plan. In short, they asked if the policy we are providing can in any way limit their ability to pay for care contained in the plan, but denied on your company's determination the care isn't medically necessary.

Please provide us with an answer so we can get back to our Employee.

Rich Mangini

++

April 26, 2006

Hi Richard. Just so I understand the question – are you asking if Aetna denies a claim for some reason can they pay for the claim out of their pocket?

J. P. Kearney

++

May 2, 2006

The employee's question appears to be simply one of, is an insured employee to look only to you (Aetna) for payment of medical procedures included in our plan. Apparently, the employee heard a state legislator say that the state protects policyholders by requiring something called the harmless clause in all hospital contracts that requires the hospitals to look only to insurance companies for payment. In essence, the state prevents hospitals from billing anyone but the insurance company for services offered by an individual's plan. The question then is, can this attempt by the state to protect the individual in any way interfere with the employee's ability to self-pay for a service Aetna might believe is unnecessary?

Rich Mangini

++

May 3, 2006

Hello Rich. If the hospital or doctor is participating in Aetna's network then they cannot bill the customer for additional charges above the Aetna payment. This is standard in all of our provider contracts. However, if Aetna concludes that a service is unnecessary then the employee can self pay with no interference from Aetna. This may be relevant if a customer has some type of cosmetic surgery.

J. P. Kearney

++

May 4, 2006

JP, Forgive me if I make sure I have this right!

I'm to tell the employee that network hospitals and doctors can only bill Aetna for services that are considered a covered service under his plan. However the employee is free to self-pay for any care Aetna concludes is unnecessary --- cosmetic surgery being a good example.

I sure hope this is right so I can get back to managing the business --- Whatever happened to the simple world I grew up in?

Rich Mangini

++

May 5, 2006
Hi Rich. Yes, that is correct. Have a great weekend.

J. P. Kearney

++

May 9, 2006
The good news is I've been able to get back to our employee. The bad news is he is upset and saying we've confirmed his worst fears. Namely, our policy unreasonably limits his access to health care.

His point is that "unnecessary care like cosmetic surgery" is not relevant here as this form of elective care is clearly outside our plan, i.e., not a covered service. As such, Aetna, by definition can't interfere with his ability to access and pay for this form of care. However, essentially all other forms of medical care are defined as "covered services" under the plan. Here, Aetna reserves the right to pre-certify the care and determine whether it is "medically necessary" in a particular situation. Consequently, if Aetna determines a covered service isn't "medically necessary" the hospitals and doctors in Aetna's network are still barred from billing the subscriber. --- If the hospital or doctor can't bill the employee, then the employee can't self pay and his access to health care is restricted. Aetna could honestly believe a covered service isn't medically necessary in a particular situation while the employee and his doctor believe just the opposite.

As I see it, there are 2 issues here. One, is the restriction on billing, as I understand it, in all Aetna's contracts with doctors and hospitals The other is a failure to disclose the restriction to our employees. On the first point, I'm not about to ask you to change your contracts. Furthermore, if I'm not mistaken, the restriction is a state requirement. There, I think we can focus on properly disclosing the issue to our employees.

Fortunately, you must have run into this problem before. Consequently, you should have some form of prepared bulletin, pamphlet or policy statement explaining the restriction that we can give our employees. In addition, I'm sure that somewhere in all the paper we got from Aetna there is an acknowledgement of the restriction. If you would provide me with both, I feel confident I can deal with this employee's concerns as well as those of any other employee he might speak to.

82

I really appreciate your help with this. The employee appears far more upset with us than Aetna as he sees us as agreeing to restrict his access to health care without telling him.

Rich Mangini

++

May 9, 2006

Hi Rich. Give me a buz this afternoon. 610-283-7036

J. P. Kearney

++

May 9, 2006

Rich Mangini Memo to Cameron's Management

I called Joe Kearney at the number he gave me. I explained that, of course cosmetic surgery would not be considered necessary in most cases. I then offered an example from my own experience where my doctor and I elected a more expensive procedure and my insurer might well have determined a less expensive alternative treatment was appropriate.

My question to Joe/Aetna, then was, "had my insurance company considered this unnecessary even though it was a "covered service", and I wanted to go ahead and pay for it myself, would I be able to?

Joe responded "yes". He said there was nothing in Aetna's policy he is aware of that would prohibit me from paying myself

Rich Mangini

.

++

May 16, 2006

JP, I've had some time to reflect on our phone conversation as well as the opportunity to reconnect with our employee. To be honest, I'm confused and a bit frustrated.

In your e-mail of May 3rd, and again on May 5th, you agreed the state requires Aetna to include language in all your contracts with doctors and hospitals that says **"they cannot bill the customer (our employee) for additional charges above the Aetna payment"** for **"any services that are considered part of his plan"**. I attaching a copy of the state regulations that, at least to my understanding, says exactly that. However, when I asked you to give me something in writing explaining Aetna's position on the restriction, you came back saying there isn't a problem and you have never heard of any such restriction.

I have to admit that when our employee first came to me, I believed he was simply misrepresenting something he heard. However, my communications with you and reading of the copy of the state regulations the employee pulled off the internet cast the issue in a whole new light. Putting it as simply as I can:

1. "Covered Services" are defined by the policy/plan.
2. The "Hold Harmless" clause in the state regulations makes it very clear hospitals and doctors cannot bill employees for "Covered Services".

3. If hospitals and doctors are not free to bill the employee, the employee cannot be free to self-pay.
4. Lastly, our company is simply asking for Aetna's published position on what is, at a minimum, a potential restriction to our employees' access to health care and a matter of public policy.

Rich Mangini

++

May 19, 2006

Hello Rich. I sent this to my contracts department so they can respond. Typically they will take several days to respond.

J. P. Kearney

++

May 25, 2006

Hi Joe, I haven't heard anything from your contracts dept. yet. Maybe you could folloe up for me. Thanks

Rich Mangini

++

May 25, 2006

Hello Rich. They advised me that the contract language simply means that the contracted provider cannot balance bill the client beyond the Aetna reimbursement. If the employee has additional questions please have him write a letter to the Aetna Grievance department. The address is PO Box 14462, Lexington KY, 40512

J. P. Kearney

Joe, I'm kind of surprised at your response.

When this subject was first raised, I honestly thought the employee had to be mistaken or have taken something out of context. It's now quite obvious the issue is real and you are doing everything you can to avoid giving us an honest answer.

Let's start with your most recent suggestion that I have our employee contact the Aetna Grievance Dept. --- That's ridiculous. The employee is only a beneficiary of our company's policy. In short, Cameron's owns the policy and it's Cameron's asking for information. Furthermore, we are only asking for Aetna's policy on what you have acknowledged is: 1.) A bar against our employees self-paying for care the policy and your contracts define as a "Covered Service", 2.) Language that is contained in all you're your provider contracts and 3.) A requirement of Pennsylvania law. --- **Are you really asking us to believe Aetna doesn't have a published policy on something this central to your operations?**

At a minimum, there have to be established guidelines for when and how a subscriber can pay for a covered service that Aetna believes isn't medically necessary, i.e., there have to be guidelines for when a provider is free to bill a subscriber. However, if the Legislature has created an insurance program that prohibits all such direct billing to a subscriber in order to protect the subscriber from any form of double billing, then it's the law and we have to accept it as fact. --- You just have to level with us.

Look, on one hand I simply want to get this issue resolved and move on. On the other hand, we are not going to short change our employees. If necessary, we will be more that willing to bring the Legislature and the Pennsylvania Insurance Department into this discussion.

Please, just level with us!   Rich Mangini

+++

June 8, 2006
Rich Mangini Memo to Cameron's Management
Joe Kearney of Aetna Insurance called today in connection with a lengthy discussion on the terms of our health insurance policy. The following points summarize our discussion on the phone:

- He apologized if his last e-mail sounded harsh.
- I said we didn't have a grievance, we just wanted information.
- He said it's a matter of interpretation. They have nothing in writing that he could send me.
- He offered to send me a copy of our contract.
- I told him I'm sure we already have a copy of our contract.
- He said if the employee still had questions he could contract the contracts dept. but he has nothing else to offer me.
- He said he was sorry but had done his best

Rich Mangini

+++

June 9, 2006
Rich Mangini Letter TO J. P. Kearney

This is to both confirm and finalize our lengthy exchange on the ability Cameron's employees to pay for health care under the terms of our Aetna policy.

1. The Hold Harmless Clause in Aetna's provider contracts forbids direct payment by a subscriber for a "Covered Service" purportedly to protect subscribers from any form of double billing.
2. "Covered Services" are defined by Aetna to be the services included in the policy benefit package and subject to Aetna's determination of medical necessity.
3. The definition of a "Covered Service" is independent of whether Aetna pays for the care or denies coverage based on medical necessity.
4. Subscribers are, however, completely free to pay for all "Non-Covered Services" which are defined by Aetna to include cosmetic care, experimental treatments and all other services not included in the policy benefit package.
5. Aetna is unable to provide a written policy, bulletin or pamphlet clarifying the impact of these contractual provisions and restrictions as requested by Cameron's
6. Our employees are to write to Aetna's grievance Department if they have any additional questions

Thank you for your time, patience and candor. It has been extremely clear this has not been an easy subject for you to discuss.

Rich Mangini

+++

June 12, 2006

Hello Rich, Once again, thanks for your business. Please feel free to reach out to me in the future if you have questions on other topics. **<u>The answer is yes to all the points in your letter (the 6 above points)</u>.** Emphasis added.

J. P. Kearney

8: <u>Blue Cross Letter to Art Hershey</u>

Please note the underlining <u>by the insurance company,</u> because it represent what appears to be a clear attempt to mislead Representative Hershey into believing subscribers are free to self-pay for care whenever Blue Cross denies coverage. A completely false conclusion. However, the wording of the letter has been so carefully chosen that the actual statements can be defended as true. I just don't think that anyone can reasonably argue this is by chance. It's far too cleverly done. And, this is from the insurer's Legislative Policy Office for the State of Pennsylvania. So if the insurer is willing to mislead one of the most senior members of the Pennsylvania Legislature, what do you think the chances are for the average subscriber to get a straight answer? --- I'll let you be the judge.

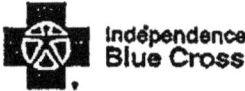

Independence Blue Cross

LEGISLATIVE POLICY OFFICE
500 NORTH THIRD STREET
SUITE 500
HARRISBURG, PA 17101

February 7, 2002

The Honorable Arthur D. Hershey
Pennsylvania House of Representatives
214 Ryan Office Building
Harrisburg, PA 17120-2020

Re: Letter from constituent Frank H. Lobb, III

Dear Representative Hershey:

This letter is in response to your request that I look into a matter raised by your constituent Frank H. Lobb, III in his letter to you dated January 6, 2002. In his letter, Mr. Lobb asked to testify before the Pennsylvania Insurance Oversight Committee regarding what appears to be Mr. Lobb's dissatisfaction with member "hold harmless" clauses in Independence Blue Cross provider contracts. Please be advised that Independence Blue Cross investigates all member complaints and we have no record of a complaint by Mr. Lobb regarding this situation. Without further detail on the provider, member and health care service involved and the circumstances Mr. Lobb encountered, and without specific consent from Mr. Lobb or the appropriate member to investigate the matter and discuss the same with you, Independence Blue Cross can offer no specific response to Mr. Lobb's concerns. However, the following general information on Independence Blue Cross' member hold harmless provisions may be helpful.

As you may be aware, Pennsylvania law mandates that a managed care plan's provider contracts contain member hold harmless provisions. These provisions are for the benefit of members. They require that contracted providers agree to look only to the health care plan for payment of covered services under the member's plan of coverage. Providers are prohibited from directly billing members for such covered services, other than allowable copayments and/or deductible amounts that are the member's responsibility under their coverage plan. This prohibition on member billing excludes billing for non-covered services, which members may receive outside of their plan coverage and for which the members are financially responsible. Any services that are not covered under a member's health insurance plan may be sought and paid for directly by our members. These provisions are contained in all Independence Blue Cross and its affiliate provider contracts for all lines of business, including traditional (indemnity) and managed care products. Independence Blue Cross and affiliates' Pennsylvania provider contracts have been filed with and approved by the Pennsylvania Departments of Insurance, for traditional (indemnity) hospital and facility contracts, and Health, for managed care provider contracts.

If you have any questions concerning the information provided in this letter, please do not hesitate calling me at (717) 233-6464.

Sincerely,

Mary-Ellen McMillen

Notes

Notes

Notes